KNACK
MAKE IT EASY

SELF-DEFENSE
FOR WOMEN

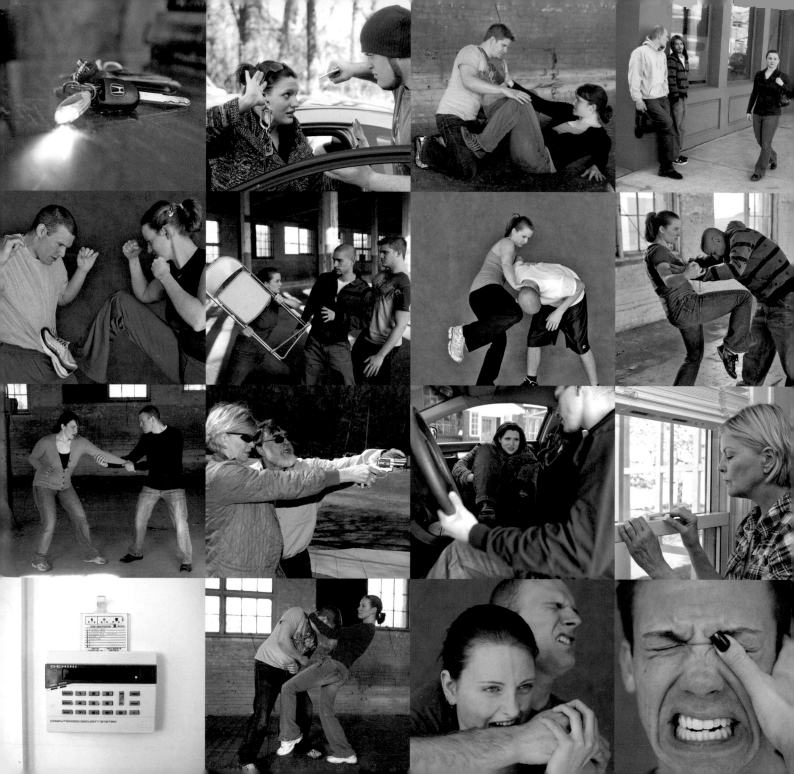

KNACK

SELF-DEFENSE FOR WOMEN

Strategies, Moves & Everyday Tactics to Gain Confidence & Stay Safe

Chris Wright-Martell

Photographs by Kristen Jensen

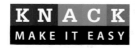

Guilford, Connecticut
An imprint of Globe Pequot Press

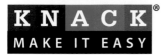

Editorial Director: Cynthia Hughes
Editor: Katie Benoit
Project Editor: Tracee Williams
Cover Design: Paul Beatrice, Bret Kerr
Interior Design: Paul Beatrice
Layout: Melissa Evarts
Cover Photos by Kristen Jensen
Interior Photos by Kristen Jensen with the exception of page 6 (right): Courtesy of Rick Ellis; page 184 (left): © Lukáš Hejtman | Dreamstime.com; and page 211 (right): © Nikolay Mamluke | Dreamstime.com.

Library of Congress Cataloging-in-Publication Data

Wright-Martell, Chris.
  Knack self-defense for women : strategies, moves & everyday tactics to gain confidence & stay safe / Chris Wright-Martell ; photographs by Kristen Jensen.
     p. cm.
  Includes index.
  ISBN 978-1-59921-956-1
  1. Self-defense for women. I. Title.
  GV1111.5.W75 2010
  613.66082—dc22
                                      2010026654

For my Dad, who makes it his priority everyday to help people

Acknowledgments

I owe deepest appreciation to Lee Lowery, Tom Allen, and Roy Harris for their guidance, encouragement, and education over the last 22 years. Thanks to my family and to my wife, Hope, for supporting my endeavors. Katie, your support and energy created a project I couldn't have imagined and carried it to fruition: thank you so much! And to my many students, colleagues, and instructors over the years, thank you for sharing your time with me.

Photographer Acknowledgments

Firstly, I would like to say thanks to everyone at Knack and to Chris and Hope Wright-Martell. This has been an amazing experience and team to work with that were both professional and fun. I'd like to thank all the models that donated their time and talents. People like Officer Libertini, Terry Hastings, Dr. Baroody, Wendy Bernard, Richard at Wooster Gun Club, the entire staff at Reliant Air, Robin Allenturner and her co-workers, and especially Melanie Vinci (for her amazing acting), Philip Rothwell (the handy-man extraordinaire), and my adorable son, Noah. ~Blessings, Kristen

CONTENTS

INTRODUCTION

The Landscape of Self-defense

I'd like to welcome you to this discussion of self-defense for women and to begin by painting you a portrait of the greater landscape.

If we imagine a timeline, with an assault or other violent crisis as the featured event, we can divide our timeline into three distinct areas: before the crisis, during the crisis, and after the crisis.

Our attention to self-defense should be divided in the same way. In the early chapters of this book you will read about preassault management, including a variety of ways in which you can improve your personal safety, as well as home, automotive, and workplace security. You will learn a variety of ways to make yourself less vulnerable to unexpected violence.

In the middle chapters you will encounter simple and effective tools that can be used during an assault when engaged in a struggle with an attacker. These tools are shown in a number of contexts, including some examples of how they might be integrated in real-life situations.

In the final chapters you will be exposed to principles of postassault management, in which the discussion focuses on the tools and relationships you will need to maintain and improve your quality of life after an assault in the short, middle, and long term.

The Hands-on Chapters

In this book I will present to you a number of tools and techniques that can be used when you are fighting for your life. These are divided into three primary categories.

The first category is techniques for the boxing and kickboxing range, when there is distance between you and your attacker. This includes skills of punching and kicking, of attacking and defending, and of moving and avoiding.

The second category of techniques addresses an area we call the "clinch range," which is when you and your attacker are holding on to each other in some fashion in an attempt to wrestle for control. The clinch range may still include punching and kicking as well as wrestling and attempting to drag the other person down to the ground.

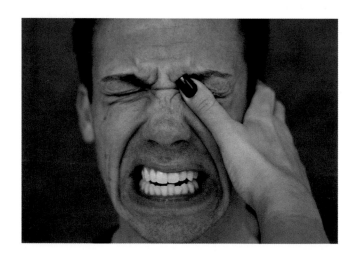

The final category of hands-on material is concerned with ground fighting, when you and your attacker are wrestling for control on the ground. Not all assault situations require these skills, but because of the relevance of sexual assault and other kinds of wrestling attacks that women face, it is critical to include them.

These three categories of training are the starting point for most hands-on self-defense training, and as such they are our primary interest here. Additional lessons are included to discuss more complex situations, including encountering weapons, facing multiple attackers, and protecting others.

The Role of the Instructor

A question emerges in self-defense training: What, exactly, is the role of the instructor?

My personal opinion, shaped by my twenty-two years in the field and training with a who's who of experts in countless martial arts, is this:

A self-defense instructor's role is to make you aware of your options and to help guide you along the path of choosing the right options for you.

The problem, in real terms, is that every individual comes to the table as a unique person with a unique situation. Each of us has our own individual body type, personality, and experiences, and these will all play a role in choosing the defense options that are best for us. We must all acknowledge our strengths, weaknesses, and limitations in order to gain the clearest picture of what we need and how we should find it.

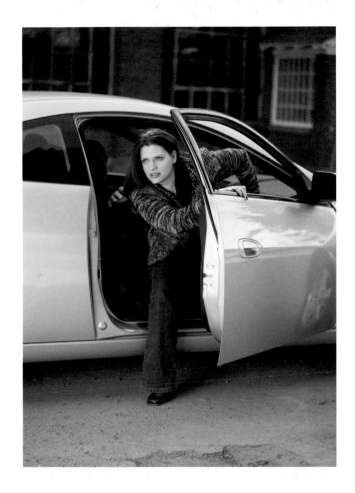

Finding the Right Answers for You

For this reason there are no universal answers in the field of self-defense. It would be a much simpler topic (and a much shorter book) if these answers existed. I could tell everyone to install a car alarm or buy a gun or kick him in the groin, and that would suffice. Unfortunately we have no such

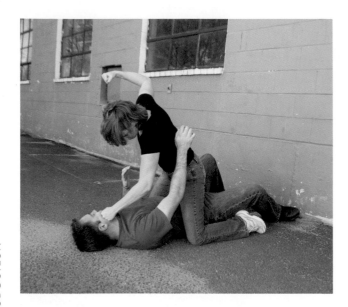

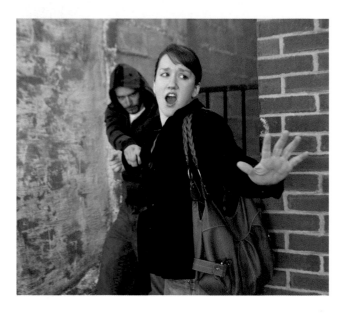

luxury. We must delve into the tricky decisions about buying a watchdog versus a guard dog, whether or not to carry pepper spray, whether we should study martial arts, and when, if ever, we should try to take a gun away from someone.

At the risk of giving away the end of the book in the introduction, I will tell you that the answers will depend entirely upon you. I will present you with options, inform you about relevant considerations, and arm you with the questions that need to be pondered, but ultimately I cannot answer many of them for you. I can tell you where to place your thumb (his eye), how to plan for a home invasion (the same way you plan for a fire), and which item you carry that hurts the most if you throw it at his face (your hot cup of coffee). I cannot, however, tell you if a home security system is right for you or if you are the kind of person who is willing to bite a stranger if your mother's safety depended on it.

How to Use This Book

This book is a catalog of options. It includes detailed analyses of broad and varied situations and presentations of options culled from over twenty martial arts. I offer you a chance to explore the tools that are available to you, to enter some deep self-analysis about your most vulnerable points, and to choose the options that will help you construct an overall plan that feels right to you.

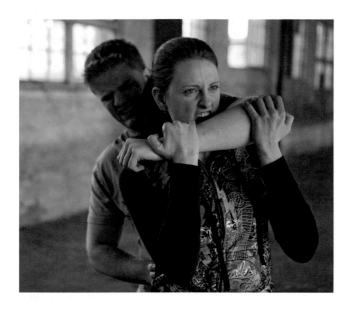

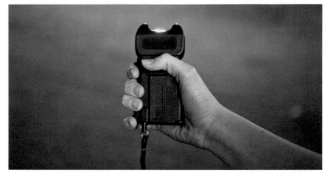

Do not assume that I have all the answers. No single instructor or resource is the final word on the matter. You are the final word on the matter. What works for someone else may not be relevant in your situation or in your life. Let this book be a launching point that helps you to explore your options and to find your answers. You will know them when they bring you a sense of security and comfort.

A Note Regarding Style

The issues, techniques, and questions presented in this book are largely applicable to both men and women of all ages. Because it has been organized and written for a female audience, it includes information and considerations voiced primarily for a female audience. Similarly, attackers in this book are written as "he," whereas defenders are almost universally "she." I do not mean any slight to the many cases of woman-on-woman violence by using this convention, nor do I intend insult to male readers who need answers to self-defense issues. As a rule, attacks perpetuated on women are overwhelmingly committed by male perpetrators, and so the pronouns were adopted for this generalization (and for the stylistic clarity when discussing both the defender and attacker).

HOME SECURITY
Begin your self-assessment by evaluating your home and exploring options to improve security

Home security is one of the most critical areas for us to explore. For most people their home is where they spend most of their time.

When we first moved into our home, my family and I sat down one night and discussed what we would do if a fire broke out in our home. We made a plan: how to call 911, how to make a safe exit, how to make a second safe exit, and so on. In making this plan, we took time to reflect on situations and limitations.

I hope that you and your family have a fire plan already. Your next task is to develop a security plan. It'll be pretty similar.

First, let's identify ways that we can make ourselves and our

Install a Security System

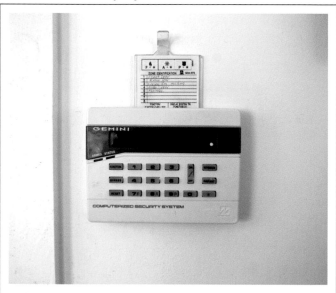

- The primary value of a home security system is that it can deter unwanted visitors. It can also alert you to possible problems and give you more time to act during a crisis.

- Home security systems come in a variety of types and prices. Some systems are monitored remotely, whereas others are controlled within your home.

- Installing a security system can give you improved peace of mind in your home.

Own a Guard Dog

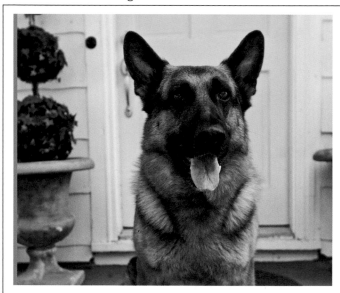

- A large (or loud) dog is another way to deter intruders.

- Watchdogs can be any size so long as they are loud and will alert you to danger.

- Some large breeds can be trained as guard dogs and will physically protect you from dangers.

- Owning a guard dog or watchdog can be expensive. It is not recommended that you bring a dog into your home solely for protection benefits.

homes less vulnerable. Look at the steps you'll want to take in a crisis: identifying the problem early, enlisting help, exiting the scene safely.

Thinking about these steps might worry you or make you feel vulnerable. Remember that we're engaged in this exercise so that you can come up with options that work for you. We don't spend our nights worrying about whether or not there will be a fire—we're comforted knowing that we have a plan that works for us. And I want you to feel the same way about your home security.

Good Locks Are Invaluable

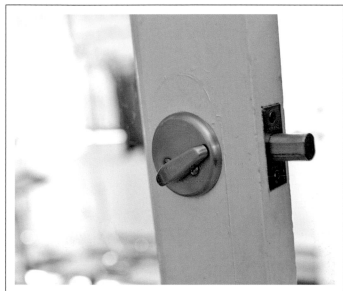

- One of the first priorities for good home security is to make sure that your house has sturdy, reliable locks on the doors and other points of entry.

- Latches and chains are not recommended. Instead, use deadbolt locks on exterior doors.

- Many locks are rated for security. Look for a grade 1 rating when choosing your locks.

- Even the best locks in the world are a waste if left unlocked. Use them.

Choose Your Neighborhood

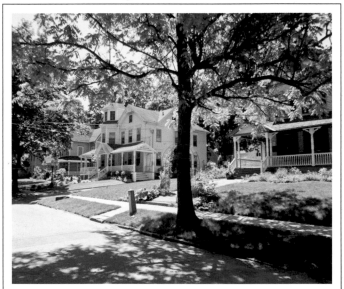

- It would be hard to overstate the importance of the area surrounding your home. The urban, suburban, or rural neighborhood you choose can make a big difference in the dangers you might encounter.

- Many Web sites and other resources can provide you with statistics about your local area or anywhere you are considering relocating.

- It's important to consider your proximity to support, including law enforcement, hospitals, and fire and rescue professionals.

AUTOMOTIVE SECURITY
Secure locations for your vehicle minimize your risk

Another place where we all spend a great deal of time is our automobile. There are some basic risks we can identify when it comes to the way we interact with our cars.

Vehicles present particular risks because the way in which we use them is predictable. Each morning we enter our car the same way when we drive to work or school or run errands. We enter and exit our vehicle so many times that we don't give it much thought, and that makes it an easy time for someone to surprise us. This is something we should keep in mind when we decide where to park at home, at work, and in the other places we visit. Minimize your risk in these transitions. And be sure to lock your vehicle, so that nobody can enter it before you do.

Presently many vehicles come equipped with safety devices, including immobilizers, loud alarms, GPS devices, panic buttons, and systems that can call an operator for assistance.

Install a Car Alarm

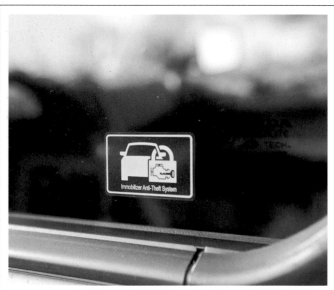

- Today's automotive alarm systems have a broad variety of features, including panic buttons, GPS locators, and voice connection with operators.

- A car alarm system can't stop a committed individual from stealing your car, but it can act as a deterrent to average thieves.

- Most importantly, a car alarm can provide access to attention and support if you are in danger.

Park in a Garage

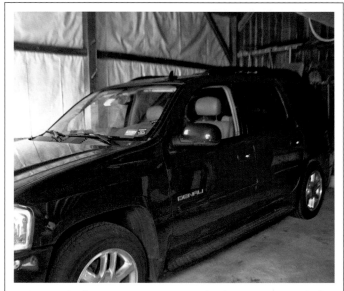

- An attached garage can provide a safe point of transition from your car to your home.

- Parking your car in a garage also reduces the opportunity for someone to hide inside your vehicle.

- Take the extra time to lock the garage door; a garage can provide an invisible entry point for intruders.

- Also be sure to securely lock the interior door between your garage and the rest of the house as an added precaution.

These tools can act as deterrents but are not something we can rely upon to prevent an assault. They can, however, give us additional options for handling a threatening situation.

Park in Safe Places

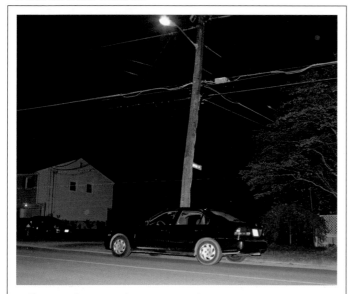

- If you park your car in an open and accessible place, it is a good idea to consider the path you will take when walking to and from your vehicle.

- Is that area well lit? Are there any obvious dangers in your path?

- Is it easy to see your vehicle? Can you see the entire path to your car?

- If you encounter trouble entering your vehicle, will others be able to see you and recognize that you need help?

Carry a Flashlight

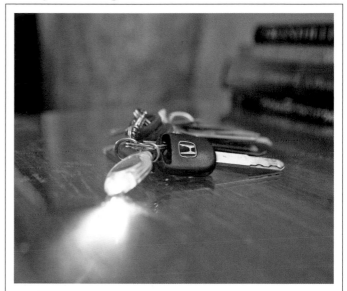

- A handy tool that is inexpensive and easily accessed is a small keychain flashlight.

- A flashlight can be helpful for mundane purposes like unlocking your vehicle in the dark and is also a prudent tool if you approach your car in a dark area.

- The ability to see your vehicle clearly can put your mind at ease or reduce the risk of your being surprised if someone or something is nearby.

WORKPLACE SECURITY

Familiarize yourself with the place where you will spend your day

If you work outside your home, your workplace is another location where you'll spend significant amounts of time. Take the time to familiarize yourself with the history, protocol, and expectations of your workplace regarding personal safety.

Almost all workplaces have an evacuation plan in case of a fire emergency and include it in employee training. This can be a good time to inquire about a similar plan for workplace violence or other kinds of crisis. If your workplace has only a

fire plan, you can often use it as your go-to crisis plan with little or no modification. It's worth learning the locations of all the exits to your building and seeing which of them could also be used as entrances. Doing this leaves you with more options if you need to evacuate quickly and also shows you all the possible places someone might use to enter.

Many schools and government-run institutions have lock-down codes that can be announced and procedures that

Know Your Workplace Exits

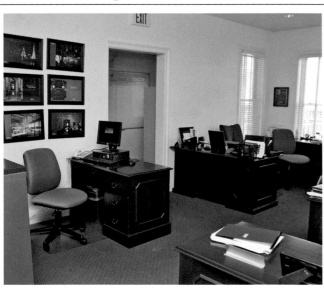

- One of the first things you should notice when you join a new workplace is the location of the exits, both routine and emergency.

- Almost all workplaces have several exits—some obvious and some that you might not think of right

away. It's worth taking the time to learn where they are and where they lead in case you ever need them.

- Remind yourself that these are potential points of exit or entry.

Garages Have Multiple Exits

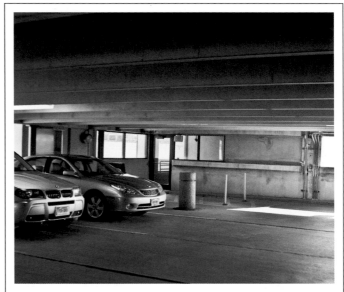

- If your workplace has a parking garage, you'll want to familiarize yourself with the entrances and exits.

- Most garages have both stairs and elevators. Knowing where to find each one can give you valuable options if you're uncomfort-

able following your usual route for any reason.

- Dark, noisy, and secluded, garages can be spooky places when you're alone. When possible, walk with someone. Try parking near a friend or coworker so you can leave together.

accompany them. Your workplace may be staffed with security personnel or have safety measures like metal detectors or alarm systems. Find out what your workplace uses. If it does not have a plan, make one for yourself, even if only informally.

You can also interview your employer about the company's past history of safety and security. If there has been any kind of incident, that's something you'll want to know. Although privacy barriers may prevent your employer from discussing specifics, find out as much as you can.

As with home and automotive security, your priority is to learn what your risks are and to find as many options as possible. From there you can select ones that are a good fit for you. Build a plan that makes you feel comfortable.

Learn Your Workplace History

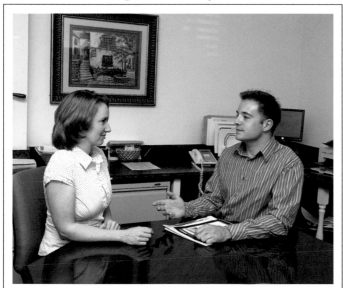

- When you enter a new workplace, discuss its security history with your superiors.

- Does this company or office have any history of violence or crisis? Have there been any incidents in the company's past? How were they handled?

- In many cases there may be no significant history of anything that may put you at risk. But knowing those answers, either way, will better prepare you for the time you spend there.

Know the Crisis Plans

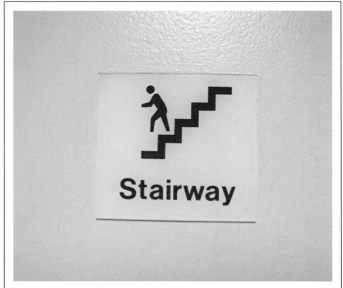

- Every workplace should have procedures for a fire evacuation. Some will also have policies for violence or other forms of crisis.

- Knowing the steps to take puts you ahead of the game. In a crisis you don't need to make a decision— you need only to act. This saves critical time when it is most needed.

- If your workplace doesn't have a plan specific to violence, use the fire plan as a starting place and modify it to suit your needs.

5

HANDS-ON TRAINING
Investigate the options for self-defense or martial arts training

We, as martial arts instructors, often speak as though everyone ought to run right out and join their local school for some training. Although this is a great option for many people, the truth is that it's not for everyone.

The benefits of training martial arts can stretch far beyond just self-defense skills. Depending on the type of classes offered, martial arts schools can provide a wide range of services to you.

Some schools focus on personal protection skills. Those schools will help you to be more aware of your environment and to give you real-world options should you ever need to fight your way out of a bad situation.

Other schools are sports oriented and will offer you an athletic training environment that will improve your physical and mental health. They may also be an excellent source of stress relief.

Self-defense Workshops

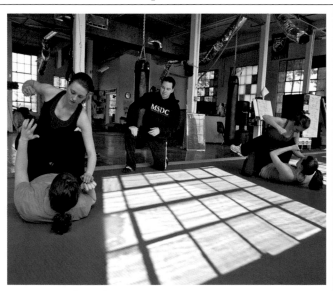

- Self-defense workshops are a good short-term source of training. Typical courses meet from one to eight sessions.

- A good workshop will introduce you to the primary areas of concern and help you find simple, effective solutions.

- Pros: Workshops like this require little commitment in the way of time and money.

- Cons: Training like this barely scratches the surface of a deep topic. Quality varies widely by instructor.

Traditional Martial Arts Training

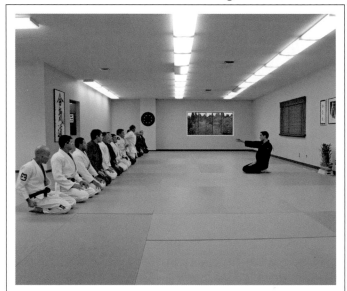

- Martial arts training is another common route for exploring self-defense. Practicing martial arts also can have benefits beyond the obvious, including improved health and fitness.

- Pros: Martial arts schools now exist in nearly every population and in such variety that you should be able to find one you like in your area.

- Cons: Every school specializes in a certain topic or type of training. A significant time commitment and financial commitment are required.

Some schools offer a traditional environment that will focus on character qualities like self-confidence, self-control, and self-discipline. They may also focus on goal setting and motivation.

Many schools will be some combination of these types of environments. Some of them build strong communities among their students and can offer a positive, social activity. Training in martial arts can be an expensive, time-consuming activity. Although it has obvious benefits, it may not be the right option for everyone.

For some people martial arts training can be inappropriate. Some people may not be comfortable knowing how to hurt someone else. Others might not be emotionally able to defend themselves physically if attacked. If you fall into one of those groups, that's okay. The real lesson is to know this about yourself and to understand that you should pursue other options to improve your safety.

Training at Home

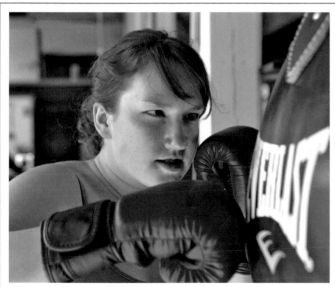

- With some experience from workshops or martial arts classes, training at home can be a great way to keep in shape and maintain your physical skills.

- Pros: It is extremely inexpensive and supremely convenient. It requires only a space to practice and minimal equipment.

- Cons: It requires a certain amount of experience to be worthwhile. Also much of the best training is done with skilled partners and trainers.

Is This Right for Me?

- Most self-defense instructors assume that hands-on training is right for everybody, but in truth it may not be for you.

- Take some time to reflect on your personality, your physical strengths, weaknesses, and limitations and then decide whether hands-on abilities would be practical skills for you.

SHOULD YOU CARRY A WEAPON?

The decision to arm yourself is a big one

One of the questions I am asked frequently is, "Should I carry a weapon?" Usually this question comes from a woman who doesn't have time to dedicate to a lot of hands-on training and wants to make sure that she feels physically secure when she's out and about. The decision is not one to be taken lightly.

The first step should be to find out what kinds of weapons and tools are legal in your community. Although some folks might want to arm themselves with anything they can—legal or not—consider the "big picture" to be your overall quality of life. If carrying an illegal weapon gets you into trouble, then it hasn't helped your quality of life. Keep that in mind when researching your options.

The next big question is, "Will I have it when I need it?" You can own all kinds of helpful tools, but if they're too cumbersome to carry around all day, you'll probably start leaving

Tasers and Stun Guns

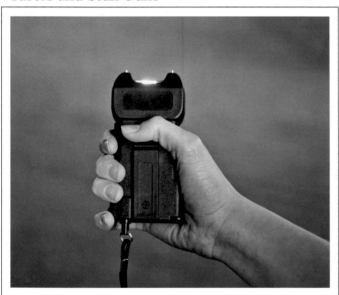

- Many self-defense devices are intended to incapacitate attackers without injury.

- These include aerosols from mace to pepper sprays and electroshock tools like Tasers and stun guns.

- The first step in deciding to own or carry a weapon is to learn what weapons are legal in your community.

- You'll also want to research the effectiveness of each option and to decide what measures you'd be willing to use. A tool you won't actually use is a liability, not an option.

Weapons without Proper Training

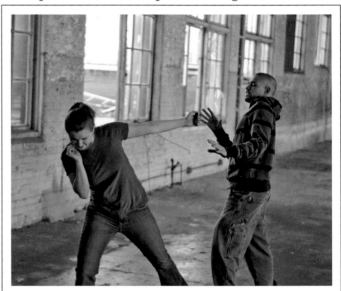

- One of the worst decisions a person can make is to carry a weapon that she isn't properly trained to use.

- Using a weapon improperly is a liability, both to yourself and any bystanders who might be around you.

- Ineffective use runs the risk of your attacker taking the weapon and using it on you. If this happens, you have armed your own assailant.

them at home, where they won't benefit you any. Rule out options that are inconvenient for you to consistently carry.

The third question is, "Will I train myself to use it appropriately?" If you have a weapon and don't receive adequate training, then your weapon is a liability. What happens if your pepper spray is taken away and used against you? What if it was a Taser, a knife, or a firearm?

The fourth question is, "Will I really use it?" Some people like the idea of having something but might not have the determination to use it on someone when it counts.

The final question is, "Can I store this appropriately so that nobody gets hurt?" Many communities require trigger locks or locked cabinets for firearms, but few require it for other personal weapons. Find a way to keep it safe.

Train with Your Weapon

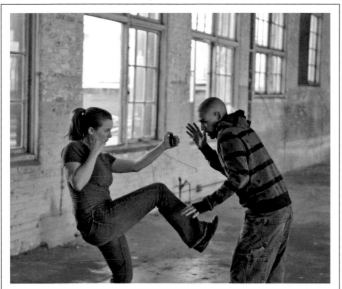

- If you decide to carry any kind of weapon, it's essential that you train with it and that in this training you integrate it with the other measures you intend to use.

- You must plan not only how to have your weapon but also how it will be used in the greater context of the situation.

- After that you must train with it as a part of your plan. Without practice it's just a theoretical skill. Put in the time.

Seek Expert Instruction

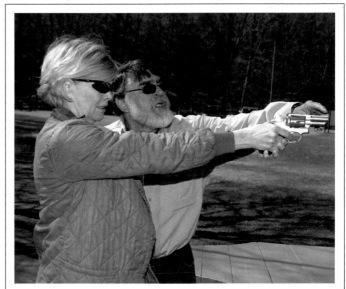

- With any weapon you should seek the highest level of instruction available.

- No matter what you arm yourself with, educate yourself about your choice.

- Learn how to use the weapon, how to store it safely, how to carry it, how to conceal it, how to deploy it, and also how *not* to do all those things.

- Learn how to disarm it. Learn how to dispose of it if you change your mind and no longer wish to own it.

YOUR RISK FACTORS

Protecting your life is about more than just fighting off bad guys

When we talk about threats, we tend to immediately focus on the external. We worry about someone breaking into our home or approaching us and threatening us. These are scary situations, and they really do happen, but that doesn't always mean that you should worry.

Sometimes our risks are much more mundane: poor diet, family history of disease, motor vehicle accidents, poisoning with household chemicals, or accidents around the home.

Although less dramatic than a personal assault, these risks are just as dangerous. In fact, depending on your situation, these may be more likely than an assault.

Healthy lifestyle choices are some of the best ways you can improve and preserve a positive quality of life.

Although many people roll their eyes at this topic, it's important to have this discussion in the context of self-defense. After all we're trying to keep you (and your quality

Maintain a Healthy Lifestyle

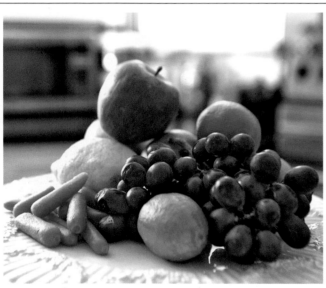

- Protecting your quality of life starts with simple decisions that many people overlook.

- The food you eat every day has the power to build a healthy mind and body or to destroy them. You choose daily to protect against disease or to encourage it.

- Find a balance that improves your quality of life overall: Find compromises that fulfill the "good for me" and also the "what I want to eat" criteria.

Home Accidents

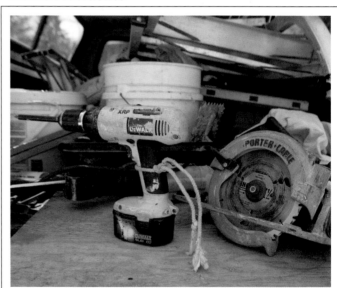

- Accidents around the home are one of the leading causes of death in the United States.

- Slips and falls, fires, suffocations, and other risks are often easily avoided but require you to take steps for prevention.

- If you're going to the trouble to defend your home from attack, be sure to safeguard your family and yourself against unnecessary risks from your home itself.

of life) safe from all threats. Shouldn't that include yourself?

As with many things, we want to strike a balance between what you want to include in your life and what you ought to include. Avoid the most unnecessary risks—store dangerous tools and chemicals appropriately, drive a little more defensively, and if you smoke, stop. Who needs an attacker if you're already endangering yourself?

· · · · · · · · · · · GREEN ● LIGHT · · · · · · · · · · · · ·

Sometimes we worry the most about external threats: other people, environmental disasters, political or economic crises. Take the time to look at your situation and see if you can create and defend a better quality of life. You may find in the end that the best peace of mind comes from a healthy diet, good exercise, and positive social activities. The best self-protection starts within you.

Store Hazardous Materials

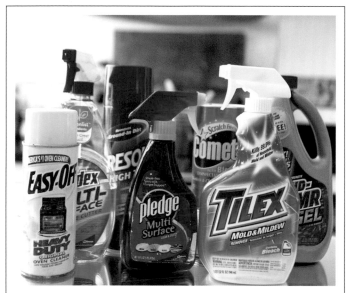

- Accidental poisonings are another leading home accident that can be fatal.

- Be aware of the potential toxins in your home. Learn how to store them safely and be sure to do it.

- Post the phone number for the local poison control center near your phone and program it into your cell phone. The national number is (800) 222-1222.

Unhealthy Choices

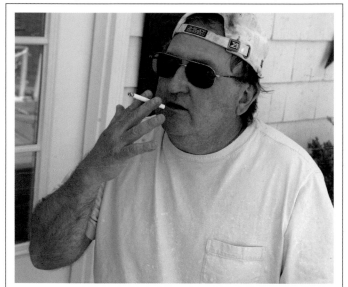

- Some people make all the right choices except for the ones that really count.

- Alcohol, tobacco, and other drugs sometimes seem to get overlooked in discussions about self-defense. In reality they could be your biggest risk factor.

- If you wouldn't take a crazy and unnecessary risk with driving or the locks on your doors or a loaded firearm, why do it with your own body?

MAKE SAFETY PLANS

Have a plan so that in a crisis you need only to act

Planning is essential. During a crisis there is no time to stop and think about what should be done—and even if there were time, we'd be so emotional that we might make irrational and unsafe decisions.

Instead take advantage of the time you have now: study your home, your car, your workplace, your family, and yourself. Look over the options you have—because you have a lot of them.

Ask yourself: "Will I improve the security measures in my home? Are there significant but inexpensive ways to do that?" (There almost always are.)

"Will I change the place where I park my car at night or at work? Will I install anything in my car or add something to my keychain or carry something in my purse that will make the walk to and from my car safer?"

Be sure to discuss and share your ideas with family, friends,

KNACK SELF-DEFENSE FOR WOMEN

Check Windows and Doors

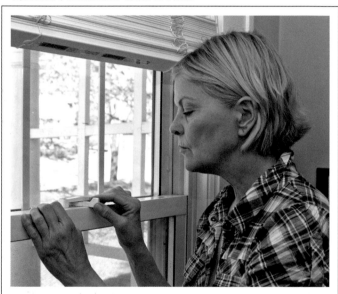

- Minimize the points of entry to your home by installing secure locking mechanisms on windows.

- Intruders look for the easiest point of entry. Be sure that windows aren't left open or unlatched.

- Glass sliding doors on the ground floor are particularly vulnerable. Be sure to install secure tracks and secondary measures like a security bar to prevent the doors from opening.

- Remember that even when difficult to open, glass windows and doors can be smashed to gain entry.

Assess Vulnerable Areas

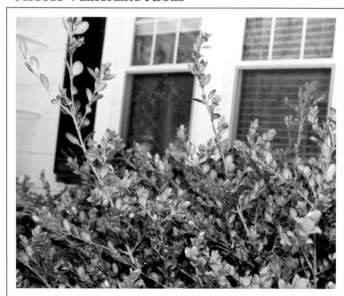

- Most intruders look for the easiest entry point that will attract the least attention.

- Look at your own home from an intruder's perspective. Ask yourself: "Where would I gain entry if I were breaking in?"

- Doors and windows that are not easily seen from the street or from nearby houses make a prime target.

- Take the time to assess, acknowledge, and fortify the areas that are the most likely targets.

roommates, and other loved ones. Solicit ideas from the people who live in your household and take into account their opinions on the plans you're forming. If you have children, use the discussion as a learning lesson about being prepared or taking personal responsibility.

Remember: Being prepared should put your mind at ease.

Discuss the Crisis Plan

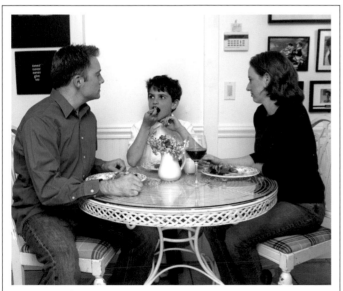

- After you've given your home a thorough assessment, it's time to create a plan.

- Be sure to take into account the limitations or needs of others who live there.

- Most households have already planned for fire

safety. Depending on your area, you might also have talked about floods, earthquakes, or other crises.

- It's not necessary to scare anyone. See this as an opportunity to teach preparedness without evoking paranoia.

Know Your Exits

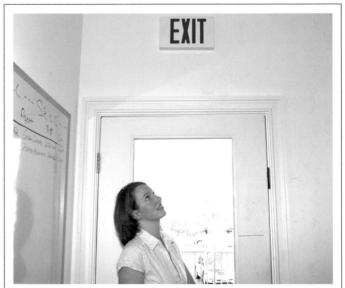

- Most people spend almost as much time at work as they spend at home.

- Knowing your environment well arms you with valuable information that allows you to assess options.

- The more "good options" you have to fall back on, the better the decisions you can make in crisis.

- Have the upper hand: Know the territory, think it through in advance, and pursue your best options.

HOME INVASION
Preventive planning can make a scary possibility more manageable

One of the scariest scenarios many people envision is that of an assailant entering their home. It's a dangerous possibility.

As we've discussed, the best thing to do now is to fortify your home in order to make it as unappealing a target as possible. If it looks like too much work (and too great a risk of being caught), most criminals will pass it by. Alarm systems, secure doors and windows, loud dogs, and a well-lit yard can be major factors in whether your home becomes a target.

Deterrents are the most important element in keeping yourself safe because they can help prevent the situation from developing in the first place.

If someone does enter your home, you'll want something to alert you right away, especially if you are sleeping. Many people choose home security systems (or watchdogs) for that very reason. After you are alerted, you can put your plan into action.

Prepared for Crisis

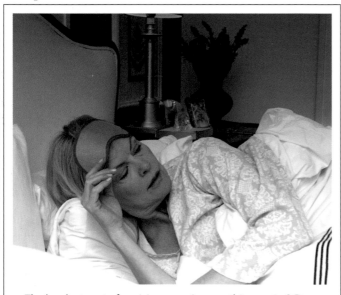

- The hardest part of a crisis can be recognizing it during the earliest stages.

- Is your alarm system or watchdog telling you that something has happened?

- Is something amiss? Does the situation not feel quite right? Go with your gut.

- Don't freeze. You have a plan. Put it into action.

Know Which Phone

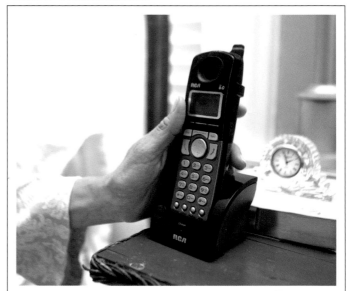

- One of the essential steps in any crisis plan is to recruit help.

- After that happens, you are not alone in this problem.

- Which phone is most accessible to your location? Is there a reliable one near the bed at all times? Where

- else might you be caught off guard?

- Is the phone a landline, cordless, or cell? Be sure to choose one that will be ready to work when you most need it.

You also want to have a method of calling for assistance. Some security systems automatically notify a support center or local law enforcement. In many cases you'll need access to a phone. Where is the closest phone? If it's a landline, will it work if the power is out? If it's a cell phone, will it have a signal? Will it be charged? If you need to evacuate the house immediately, is there a phone you can take with you? Where is it?

If you live with others, be sure you'll have a method of alerting them and helping them put the plan into action. If it's safe to do so, evacuate everyone from the house. Plan multiple exits in case some are unsafe.

It is not recommended to confront the intruder(s). You don't know who these people are, what they're armed with, and what they're capable of. It's better to avoid them at all costs.

Help Others

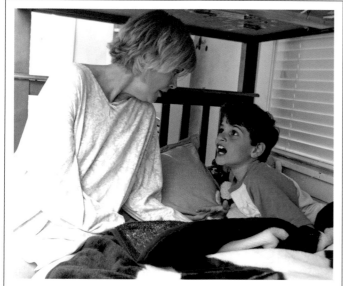

- If you live with other folks, the next step of the plan will most likely be to make them aware of the danger.

- It may be necessary to do this quietly and discreetly to avoid attracting attention from your intruder(s).

- This is when the household discussion pays its dividends: There is little time now to discuss anything. When everyone knows his or her role, you can all move quickly.

Plan Multiple Exits

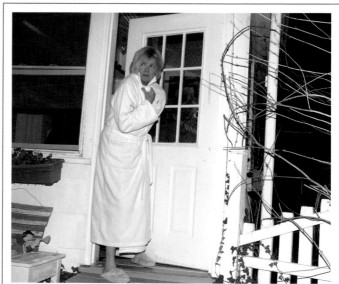

- If you feel it is safe to evacuate your home, do so.

- Plan multiple exit points, just as you would for a fire.

- Doing this provides you with valuable options. If danger prevents you from using your preferred exit, having backup exits will prevent your plan from stalling.

- Just as with entry points, exit points may not always be obvious at first. Look at windows, doors, and any other possibilities.

GO SOMEWHERE SAFE

The plan doesn't end when you safely exit your home

Most people when frightened try to get away from the danger. But "away" isn't a destination by itself. Your plan should have a final goal: Where will you go?

In urban and suburban communities, you may have the option of going to a neighbor's house for safety. If someone you know and trust lives nearby, you can designate his house as a safe destination. Be sure to discuss this with the person ahead of time; a crisis in the middle of the night is not when you want to have an extended discussion on his front doorstep.

If you live in a more remote area, you might prefer the option of creating a safe place to hide and barricade yourself if you need to leave your home. Creating a hidden shelter on your property is one way to provide yourself with a safe haven.

If you'll have access to your vehicle, you can select

A Safe Neighbor

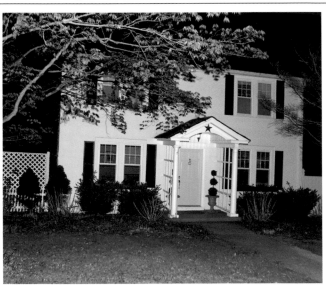

- Having a neighbor you trust and can depend upon is a great asset.

- A safe location nearby brings tremendous assets to the situation: more people, medical supplies (if needed), phone access, and additional locked doors and other barriers between you and your assailant.

- Don't forget to include your neighbors in the discussion of your plans.

- In return your home can be the safe destination for your neighbors in their own crisis plans.

Bring Your Keys

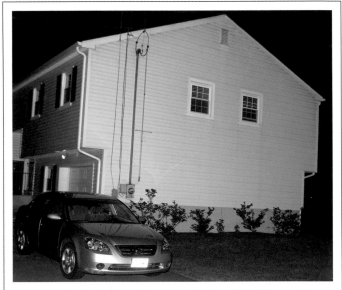

- If your vehicle is accessible when you exit your house, make sure to bring your keys.

- This means that you will need to leave your keys (or duplicates) along the path to your exit—make sure this is built into your plan.

- Having the ability to drive away from the scene gives you additional freedom and the opportunity to reach a safe destination.

- If you can build this into your plan, do it.

destinations that are farther away. Family and friends might offer a safe, supportive environment. It's also good to know the nearest locations where you can find twenty-four-hour law enforcement and medical attention.

Lastly, consider seasonal issues. If you're escaping in sleepwear, don't plan to spend hours hiding outside in winter if you live in a colder climate.

Other Safe Destinations

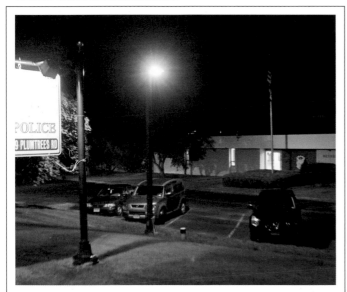

- If a neighbor's house is not accessible, or if you are able to drive off instead of simply walking, there are other locations you can seek for help.

- Police stations are an obvious choice for protection.

- Fire stations are also a good place to seek assistance, including first aid.

- Hospitals are another good destination, not only because of the availability of medical attention but also because they are often guarded by security staff twenty-four hours a day.

What Is My Plan?

- Review the options regarding home safety. Decide what your biggest concerns are.

- Take an honest look at your situation. Discuss it with family and friends.

- Create a plan. It doesn't need to be perfect, but it needs to work for you.

- Take steps to make implementing your plan easier. Fortify your home, if need be.

DANGEROUS PLACES & SITUATIONS

Recognize when your environment puts you at unnecessary risk

Your surroundings can put you at risk in two major ways: They can expose you to harm, and they can remove your access to support. It's important to avoid situations that do either of these and especially the ones that do both.

Take notice of your surroundings, especially when you are somewhere unfamiliar. Make note of any obvious dangers or concerns. Is there anything inherently dangerous? Are there people around? Do you know them? What can you observe about them instantly? Are any exits available to you? Where will they take you? Where would you need to go in an emergency?

As always, these questions aren't asked to worry you. Take the moment to observe, to evaluate, and to make quiet internal decisions. And then take a breath because you've got it covered. If your quick assessment tells you that you can relax now, then do so. If not, keep your eyes sharp but

Urban Locations

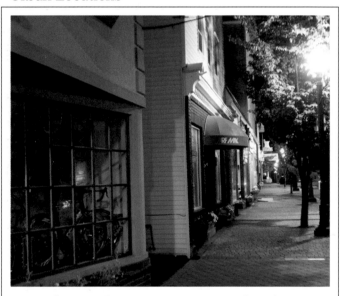

- In city locations threats can emerge from every doorway and alleyway.

- Your awareness level is your biggest asset in busy areas. Learn to distinguish genuine threats.

- Be aware of your location and the people around you. Don't become paranoid; you don't need to worry at all times. Maintain an attitude of "paying attention" without being afraid.

Rural Locations

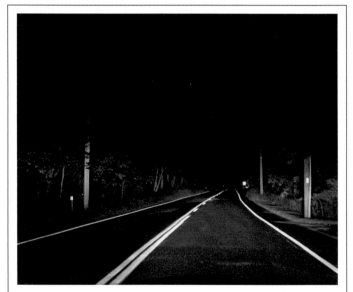

- The dangers of rural locations are the opposite of urban ones: Lack of access to other people and support is a primary concern.

- Areas may not be well lit, be within earshot of other people, or have cell phone reception.

- Rural areas may be many miles from hospitals, law enforcement, fuel, supplies, or other aid.

- Avoid isolation in unfamiliar, remote areas. Make provisions for communication and supplies in case you need them.

try not to get too worked up. You'll want to be calm, cool, and collected if you need to navigate a tricky situation.

Keep in mind the two goals you want to manage: avoiding danger and having access to support. If it looks like you might be headed for a dangerous situation, take stock of your ability to call for help. This could be making a quick exit, yelling to anyone nearby, using a nearby phone (or your cell, if you have service), sounding a personal siren or whistle, pulling a building fire alarm, blowing a car horn, or doing anything else you can do to bring help to you.

Most women have a great intuition for when things "just don't feel right." Listen to that intuition. If the hairs on the back of your neck are up, go with your instinct. And if it tells you to leave, leave.

Forced Isolation

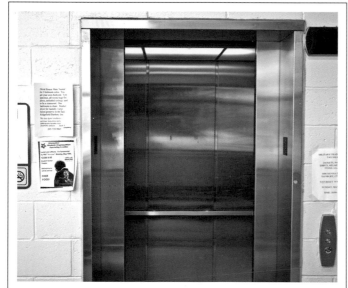

- Sometimes situations force you into isolation. When possible, find alternatives to these situations.

- If you must enter these situations, there's no need to panic. Stay relaxed and be aware of what goes on around you. Notice the people around you and take note of strange behavior.

- Don't be alarmed unless something tells you to be alarmed.

Crowded Places

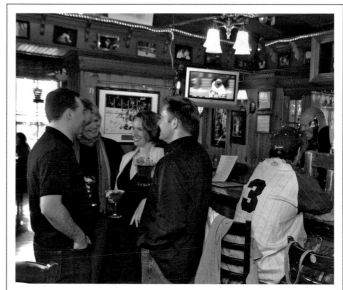

- Sometimes isolation occurs in crowded places. You may find yourself surrounded by people whom you don't know or who make you uncomfortable.

- In these situations familiarize yourself with your options. Can you leave if you need to? Are people— employees perhaps—present who could assist you?

- Taking a moment to assess your situation and to note your options can help calm you in moments of turmoil. It can also alert you to any trouble signs that you may have overlooked.

PARTIES

Take a few simple precautions to help avoid potential problems

If you're a member of social circles that have parties, some specific risks are wise to manage.

There's a big difference between parties with and without drinking. Alcohol (or any other judgment-altering substances) can make a world of difference in your behavior as well as the behavior of the people around you. If you can't think perfectly clearly—and neither can your companions—risks are greatly increased.

One of the major decisions to be made is how you'll leave the party. Will you be driving? Hitching a ride with someone else? Walking? Staying over? Plan this ahead of time, especially if you're drinking.

You'll also want a backup method of leaving if something happens and you need to leave *now*. You might consider having a second designated driver or a means of accessing public transportation. You could store the number of the

Partying and Drinking

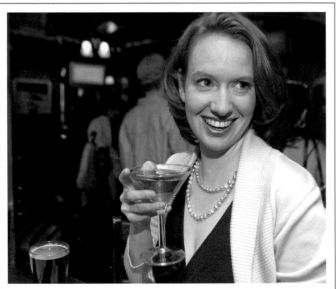

- Make some decisions before you head to the party. The first question should be, "Will I be drinking at the party?"

- Be honest with yourself. Don't tell yourself that you'll go but not drink if that isn't a reasonable option for you.

- If drinking at the party will lead to trouble, decide whether you should go. Don't just assume it'll work itself out.

Plan a Ride

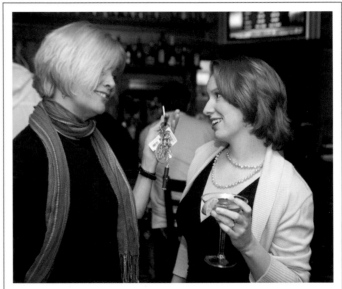

- The second question has two versions. The first is, "How will I get home, assuming that things go as planned?" If you drink, who is driving?

- The second is, "How will I get home if there's a problem, and I need to leave early?" If something

happens, and you need to make an exit, what is your option?

- Some situations can leave you in a tight spot if you have to wait for someone (including yourself) to sober up.

local taxi service in your cell phone or call another friend who could come and get you.

Party situations, especially ones with alcohol, are a prime environment for sexual assault. Intoxication leads to poor judgment on all sides, even among friends or coworkers. Whether it stems from a drunken miscommunication or an intentional predatory attack, the risk of these events is exacerbated by lowered inhibitions and impaired judgment.

In view of all these concerns, exercise responsibility. If you can't drink without becoming overwhelmingly intoxicated, then some situations are wrong for drinking. If you can't go to that party without drinking excessively, then sometimes it's better if you miss that party.

Let's be clear: The message isn't to not go to parties or drink at parties but instead to follow this motto: "A little bit of planning avoids a lot of unnecessary problems."

Know Your Companions

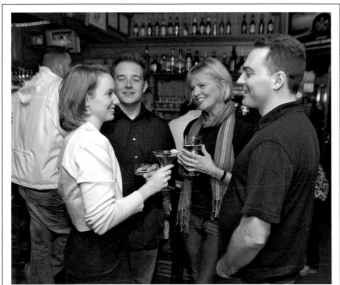

- When alcohol is involved, it's best to be surrounded by people you know and trust.

- Having friends there who will watch out for your well-being is supremely valuable.

- Avoid being left alone without any support, especially among strangers.

- Exercise good judgment even among people you know: The majority of assaults, especially sexual assaults (roughly 75 percent), are committed by someone the victim knew.

Assessment versus Blame

- Sometimes we assess our decisions afterward to look for better ways to handle events.

- Doing this is NOT the same as blaming ourselves for the decisions we made.

- Recognize that in any situation, you make the best decision you can with the information you have.

- Be okay with that afterward.

GIVE YOURSELF THE ADVANTAGE

Identify your personal strengths and weaknesses and acknowledge them as you plan

People come in all shapes and sizes, in all types of personalities, and have all kinds of experiences. Spend a little time getting to know yourself from a self-defense perspective in order to better choose the best options for your safety.

For starters, what is your body type? Are you tall and lanky? Short and compact? Somewhere in the middle? Do you carry more of your strength in your legs or in your arms? If you had to choose one, are you faster or stronger?

Do you have a background in any kind of athletics? Have you ever played any sports that involve running? That's a valuable skill to have for self-defense. What about swinging a stick or a racket? If you were holding a stick now, could

Every Body Has Advantages

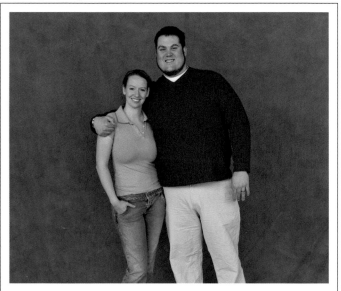

- Appraise your body type. Are you tall? Short? Somewhere in the middle? What is your fitness level? You aren't judging your body to be "good" or "bad" but instead looking at strengths.

- Tall people have a reach advantage that serves them well in punching and kicking.

- Shorter, more compact body types can be harder to wrestle against. Whereas men carry much of their strength in their upper body, women have better strength and flexibility through the hips and core.

Fitness Is a Factor

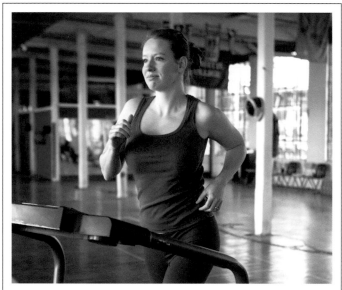

- When planning for most crisis situations, one of the most valuable skills is the ability to escape.

- This begs the question: How far can you run and at what speed? How tired would that leave you?

- What if you needed to climb over or under something? Could you do that?

- How hard could you hit somebody if you had to?

- Being physically fit can open up new options for dealing with a crisis.

22

you hit somebody pretty hard with it? Did you ever play any sports that involved pushing, checking, or tackling people?

Take an honest look at yourself. Do you have any relevant limitations? For example, if I were on crutches with a broken leg, I wouldn't make self-defense plans that revolve around my ability to run away. Instead, I might favor plans that involve hitting people with my crutches and always carrying my cell phone in order to summon help. Do you have any short-term or long-term limitations that need to be considered?

Your personality is another factor. Are you a take-charge, take-action kind of person? Do you shy away from conflict? Do you have trouble speaking your mind? Do you have trouble backing down from a challenge? None of these personalities is wrong or bad for self-defense, but to have the best options in place, you should know yourself well.

If you're someone who can't bring yourself to hit another person, make thorough plans so that you're never stuck with hitting as your only option.

Personality Matters

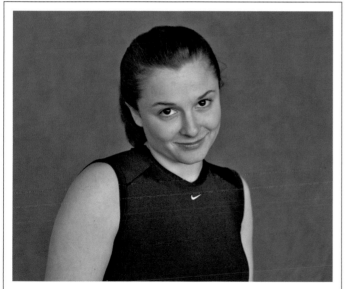

- Some people have take-charge kinds of personalities. They make decisions and put them into action.

- Others are more shy or reserved. Or they prefer to think over all of their options before acting.

- Different plans require different levels of boldness. Some people might be willing to make a public scene to attract attention, whereas others would hesitate. Which are you?

- Reflect on your personality type when deciding what options are realistic for you.

You Have Skills

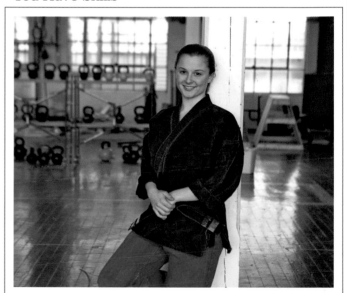

- All of us have some life experiences, skills, or training of some kind. Whereas some skills like martial arts training apply to self-defense in obvious ways, plenty of other traits are superbly valuable.

- Do you make friends well? Speak in a way that influ-ences people? Win people over? Are you chatty?

- Do you remember faces? Names? Dates? Numbers? Stories?

- Do you think quickly under stress? Do you make quick mental calculations? Do you think laterally?

23

THE WORLD AROUND YOU

Observe what's happening instead of tuning it out

In today's world we split our focus among many things at once. Multitasking is now a way of life, and we spend our time in a state of partial attention.

Although no single thing is responsible for this shift, much of our divided attention is encouraged by portable technologies. Most cell phones today can act as miniature versions of full computers, offering not only calls and text messages but also e-mail, weather, news, directions, movie times, and general Internet browsing. Personal music players have become even more widespread than in previous decades and so supremely portable that we can use them everywhere.

And even when our electronics are switched off, we find ourselves so wrapped up in our own thoughts and hectic schedules that we often pass through our environments without even noticing them.

Cell Phone Use

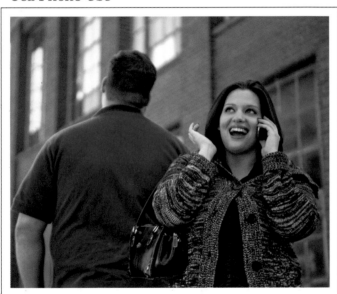

- Too many people wrap themselves up in their cell phone conversation and become oblivious to their surroundings.

- Limit your cell phone use when in public areas—not only because it's polite but also because you may need to pay better attention to your surroundings.

- Engrossing yourself in a cell phone conversation can also be a dangerous clue to predatory individuals nearby that you aren't paying full attention to what's happening around you.

Noise Insulation

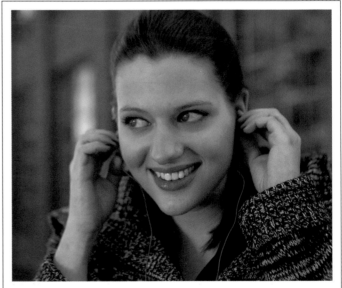

- In recent years it has become even easier to wear a portable audio device while running or cycling. Although it's enjoyable, it can also be dangerous.

- Hearing is one of the primary senses we use to detect danger. Shutting out that information could mean that you don't hear an oncoming car or an approaching individual.

- Headphones also communicate vulnerability to predators: Headphones are a visual sign that you are not listening.

For the sake of your own safety, it's time to make an effort to change all that.

As you move through your day, take note of the world around you. How far does your own awareness extend? Is it the same indoors and outdoors? Is it different when you're driving? How about when you're on the phone? When you watch TV? When you're writing an e-mail? Sending a text message? Carrying groceries?

How Do You Walk?

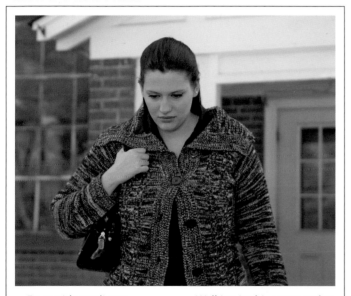

- Even without distractions, some people do not engage their environment.

- Walking with your head down is a conscious choice not to observe what's happening around you.

- Walking in this manner also communicates vulnerability and submissiveness, exactly the message that an attacker hopes to find. We'll discuss this more in the next few pages.

Impaired Peripheral Vision

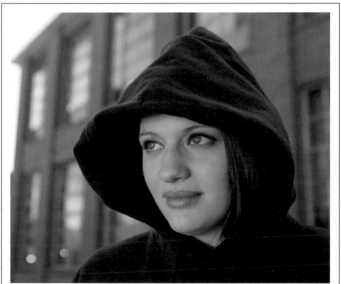

- Some hats, hairstyles, scarves, sunglasses, and hoods can severely limit peripheral vision, making it harder to see your surroundings.

- Other clothing decisions can communicate obliviousness to safety: Plenty of skirts (and high heels) make walking quickly or running an impossibility.

- Let's be clear on the message here: It's not that you shouldn't go out wearing your favorite cute shoes—just be aware of the consequences that your choices can have.

25

YOUR OWN BODY LANGUAGE
What messages are you sending to others?

Your body language communicates a great deal to the people around you. It sends out constant messages on your behalf.

People who prey upon others pay close attention to the body language of their potential targets. They're often looking for someone who is already in a victim mind-set: low self-confidence, poor self-esteem. Those qualities can be signs of an easy target—someone who is unlikely to fight back. Predators look for the easy target because it's low risk for them.

Portraying weakness and signs of low self-confidence attracts predators. What body language communicates this? Slumped shoulders, the inability to look someone in the eye, a weak frame, and a tired or timid expression are all signs of low self-confidence. Outward signs of illness can also communicate vulnerability: coughing excessively, having difficulty breathing, walking with a limp.

On the other end of the spectrum, some people

Lacking Confidence

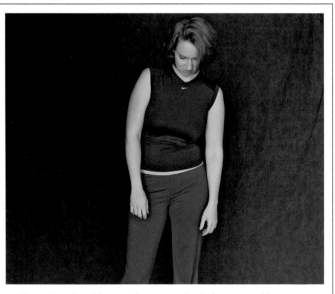

- Slumping shoulders and a collapsed torso are big clues to body language that lacks confidence.

- Downturned eyes suggest an inability to meet others' gaze. This is another big communicator of insecurity.

- Body language like this looks deflated and defeated. It says, "I've given up."

- "I'm a victim already" is definitely NOT the message you want to broadcast to would-be attackers.

Looking Aggressive

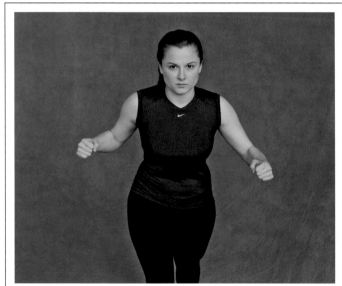

- Note the tension in the hands and face here as well as the puffed-out chest.

- This body language is particularly aggressive: The message is, "Go ahead, challenge me. I dare you."

- You might think that this is a better message to send

than that of the photo to the left, but it may not be. Aggressiveness is often a sign of insecurity, especially if it seems phony.

- Additionally, aggression rarely makes for a good social attitude. Instead, something sincere and maintainable is needed.

communicate far too much confidence. It is often interpreted by other people as aggression: wide eyes, tensed muscles, encroachment of others' personal space, a loud voice. People who are overly aggressive tend to puff themselves up and stand as tall as they can, dominating the visual scene. Although this kind of message can sometimes deter predatory types, others are savvy enough to know when it is genuine and when it is an act. Some people with over-the-top aggressive body language behave in this way to try to cover up low self-confidence and will fold in the face of a real threat. Expert predators can often spot the difference.

The ideal level of body language for self-defense is one that communicates healthy confidence. It is assertive without being aggressive and shows that you are alert and aware. It sends the message that you pay attention to your environment and respond to it appropriately.

Confidence and Assertiveness

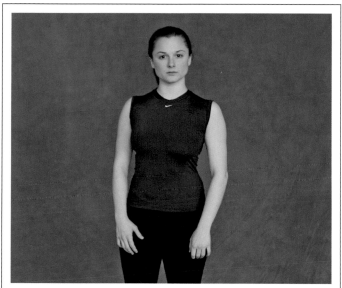

- Confidence is most notably marked by an upright posture. A person with confidence stands tall.

- Confidence is also shown by visual engagement: A confident person is not afraid to look at her surroundings or at other people.

- It's important to appear assertive in these ways without the tension bred by aggression. Calm, steadiness, and resolution are what you want to communicate while being engaged in your environment.

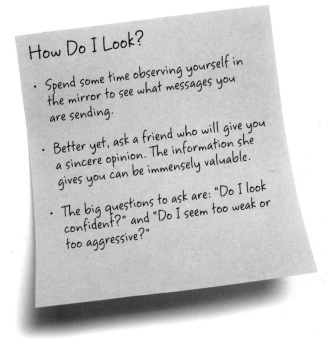

How Do I Look?

- Spend some time observing yourself in the mirror to see what messages you are sending.

- Better yet, ask a friend who will give you a sincere opinion. The information she gives you can be immensely valuable.

- The big questions to ask are: "Do I look confident?" and "Do I seem too weak or too aggressive?"

ACCESS TO SUPPORT

Is your cell phone ready to help you when you need it?

Cell phones are nearly universal now. These handy conveniences can be a useful tool for personal protection because they can bring the world to your location at the touch of a button, no matter how remote.

The first thing to do is to store your local emergency numbers into your phone, so that you will have them at your fingertips if you need them.

Even without stored numbers, your phone needs to meet

four criteria to be useful to you: It needs to be charged, it needs to work properly, it needs reception, and you need to know where it is.

These four may sound obvious, but take a moment to reflect. How often does your phone run out of power while you're out and about? A dead phone is no help.

Similarly, some people continue to use a broken phone rather than pay to replace it. If your phone has limited

Store Emergency Numbers

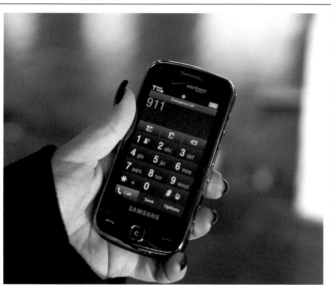

- Storing emergency phone numbers in your cell phone is a good way to have quick access to them in an emergency.

- Here are some numbers that are wise to store:

- Store your local police department, both emer-

gency (911) and nonemergency dispatch numbers.

- Include your doctor, the nearest hospital, and the poison control center.

- Store the number for emergency roadside assistance if you subscribe to a service.

In Case of Emergency

- The acronym ICE (In Case of Emergency) is now a common entry containing personal contact info in cell phones.

- Rescue workers are now trained to check cell phones on patients to see if they have an entry labeled "ICE."

- This is a good entry to use for the contact info of a loved one as well as any important medical information about yourself.

function because it had an accident, replace it. You want a phone you can rely on when it is needed.

Don't skimp when it comes to your phone service. If your phone often has trouble connecting in the places where you spend time, it won't be much help to you. Find a carrier and a plan that offer the best reception in the places where you're likely to be.

Most importantly, know where your phone is. Consider attaching a phone clip to your purse or belt. You may not have the time to look for your phone in a crisis. Plan ahead.

Another growing use of cell phones for self-protection is for storage of your emergency contact info and any important medical info in an entry labeled "ICE." "ICE" stands for "In Case of Emergency," and rescue workers are now trained to look for such an entry if they find someone in need of help.

Cellular Reception

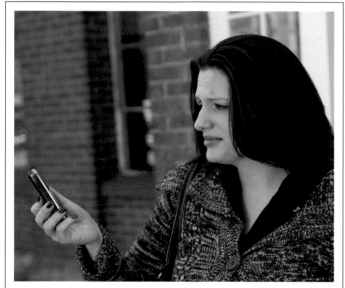

- A cell phone is only as good as its reception. If your cell phone is a part of your emergency action plan, you should subscribe to the service carrier with the best reception in the areas where you spend time.

- If your phone is unable to provide service in the places where you might need it (home, work, other common locations), it becomes a liability. Consider changing your service plan (or your crisis plan) if this happens.

Where Is Your Phone?

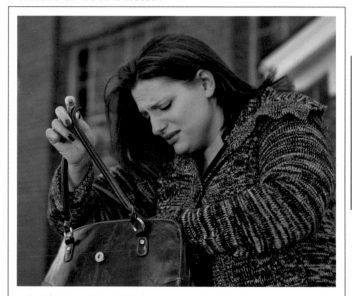

- Deployment is a critical issue with any tool that you may need in a crisis.

- If you carried a weapon and suddenly needed it, you wouldn't want it buried somewhere in the bottom of your purse. The same rings true for your phone.

- Consider keeping your cell phone in a holster on the outside of your purse or in an easily accessible pocket on your clothing.

UNWANTED ATTENTION
Notice when others take too much interest

Now that you're paying more attention to what's happening around you, it's time to see who is paying attention to you.

Someone can pay you unexpected attention for a wide range of reasons, from completely harmless to completely sinister. Before we can read his intentions, we need to be aware of the attention to begin with.

If someone is looking at you, that's an obvious sign he's paying attention. If you notice it, see if it's a quick glance or a persistent gaze. Is he staring? Does he look away, guilty, if your eyes meet his? Does he hold your gaze and look intimidating? Is he trying to attract your attention or avoid it?

Many people, however, train their eyes to deceive others. They can appear not to be looking at you, and yet they are still paying attention. What gives it away? The rest of the body.

Most people turn their torso to face the thing that's on their mind. Some people also do this with their feet. If someone

Who Is Watching?

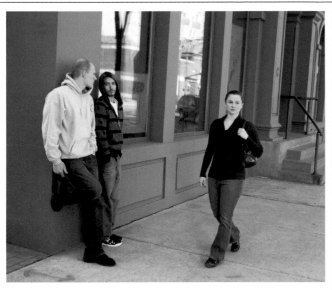

- The men in this picture are pretending not to pay attention by turning their heads toward each other as the young lady passes by.

- However, their real intentions are shown by the torso and feet, which are all pointing toward her.

- The message from the men's body language is clear: She is the focus of their attention. Don't be fooled by the direction they're facing.

Being Followed 1

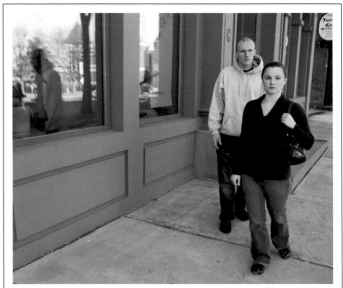

- What should you do if someone follows you?

- First you need to notice that it's happening. When walking, take the opportunity at corners or other stopping points to see who's around you.

- If you're not sure whether someone is intentionally following you, observe his body language, especially when he knows you are watching him.

- You can also watch him in a less obvious way by looking in a reflective surface such as a store window.

is looking away with his face or eyes but has his upper body pointed directly at you, he may actually be paying more mind to you.

As an exercise, watch people in conversation. You can often judge how interested someone is by where he turns his torso.

MAKE IT EASY

A frequently asked question is this: "Where should I go if I'm walking and someone is following me?" For starters, avoid going somewhere isolated or private. Instead, head for a crowd. Go somewhere busy. As for the person following you, turn around and address him. Be loud and firm. "Hey! I don't know you. You need to stop following me." Say it so everyone hears you.

Being Followed 2

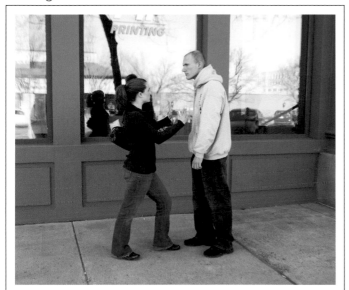

- The easiest way to deal with someone who may be following you is to address him.

- If you feel threatened, one good option is to address the threat directly. Turn your body to face the person fully and speak loudly and confidently: "You need to stop following me."

- The more people who hear you, the better.

- Don't add an "or else I'll . . ." consequence to your statement—it takes the punch out of it. Be firm. Use the tone of voice you would for a naughty puppy.

Followed in Your Car

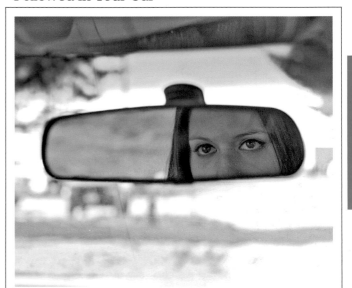

- When driving, you can also pay attention to the cars behind you.

- If you notice a car that appears to be following you, pull into a well-populated, well-lit area. Don't turn off your engine. If the other car pulls over, too, leave the area. See if the car follows.

- If you become concerned that the car is, in fact, following you, proceed directly to a safe location: police station, hospital, and so forth.

31

AGGRESSIVE BODY LANGUAGE
Recognize visual cues that display aggression and hostility

Reading hostile body language is an important skill. Agitation and hostility are key precursors to violence. If we can successfully see these early warning signs, we can respond sooner, before the situation gets more out of hand.

The biggest indicators of aggression are tension in the face and limbs, rapid movement, and loud speech or noises. When we anticipate conflict, the body reacts with the release of adrenaline, which is responsible for our "fight or flight"

instincts. Pupils dilate, expecting to need narrow, heightened vision. Blood flow increases in preparation for action. This is why some people become red in the face, or the vein in their forehead becomes prominent.

Many times people show tension in their jaw, forehead, or hands and arms. The tension can show itself in flexing muscles, furrowing eyebrows, or clenched fists. These indicators let you know that the person is becoming enraged.

Clenched Jaw

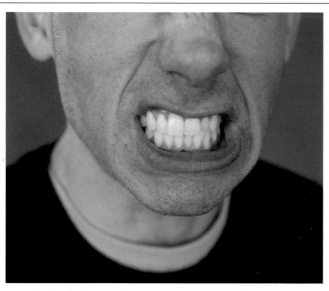

- A clenched jaw muscle is a common sign of aggression and anger.
- This can also be accompanied by pursed lips. The tension around the mouth is evident.

Clenched Hands

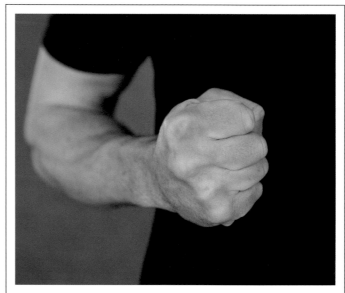

- A clenching of the hands is an indication that this person is hostile.
- The person may be visualizing violent actions or simply clenching his hands in an unconscious gesture.

Often people who are becoming aggressive will use large, abrupt movements with their arms or body. This is an indicator of their excitement and agitation. Large movements, especially those overhead, make a person appear bigger—humans do this to suggest dominance, just as some other animals do.

Throbbing Forehead Vein

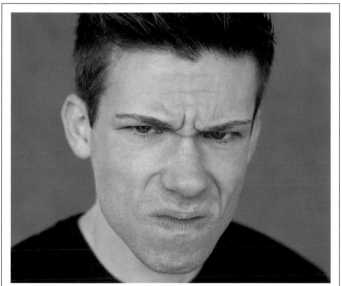

- Many people show an increased blood flow to their face when angered.

- This can show with a throbbing of a forehead vein, reddening of the face, widening of the eyes, and dilation of the pupils.

- Additionally, the eyebrows often move inward and downward as an expression of anger.

Large Gestures

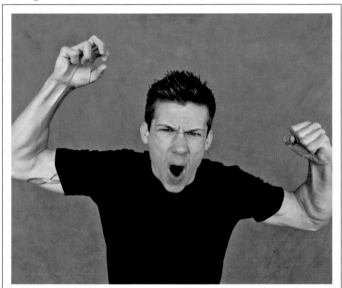

- Large, sweeping gestures can be a sign of boiling hostility, especially when made overhead or toward someone.

- These gestures are primal expressions of aggression and dominance.

- These gestures may also be jerky or abrupt, which further shows anger.

AWARE & ALERT

33

DECIDING TO ACT
Early action is best, and it can take many forms

When a situation is clearly hostile, act as quickly as you can. The earlier you intercede, the better.

The tricky aspect of violent attacks is that we don't get any warning or any choice in the matter. We don't choose the time, place, or person(s) involved. It could be at the worst time for us, when we're busy and not feeling well and not paying attention and need to be somewhere else.

As for the attacker, we don't know much about this person.

We don't know his physical, mental, or emotional state. We don't know his criminal, medical, or psychiatric history. We don't know what he can or will do. We don't know what he is armed with or what diseases he carries. We don't know who else in the area might be on his side.

With all these factors stacked against us, we need to act before more things leave our control. Our action needs to be quick and effective. It should resolve the situation.

Disengage

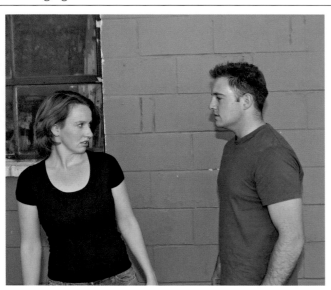

- Sometimes the best action to take is to leave the scene.

- When you realize that a situation is headed for violence, one way to defuse the situation is to leave it entirely.

- When you see that the situation is going to become physical, don't wait. Leave immediately.

- Don't worry about appearances or the impression it will make. These can be explained later. What's important now is your safety.

Speak Up

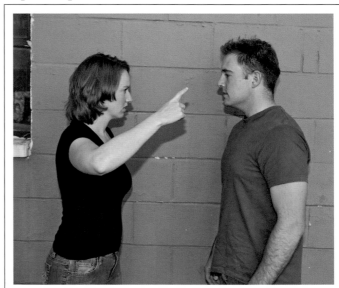

- Another way to intercede before action becomes physical is to speak up.

- Verbal intervention takes a variety of forms, from gentle deescalation to more direct, assertive approaches.

- The verbal strategies you use depend a great deal on the situation and on your personality. Some people struggle to be assertive with strangers or in stressful situations.

The action you take will depend on your self-assessments and the options you've made available to yourself. It might be escaping, verbally deescalating, defending yourself physically, deploying a weapon, or even striking first.

Defending against Aggression

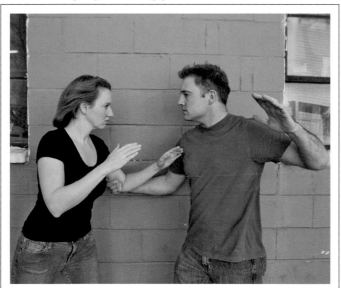

- If the situation has progressed to a physical altercation, then physical defenses become an appropriate choice.

- Physical defenses may be simply a way of halting an incoming grab, hit, or choke. More likely they may also include countermea-sures that control or injure your assailant.

- If you have received physical training in any martial arts or other hands-on approaches, this is where you will need it.

Striking First

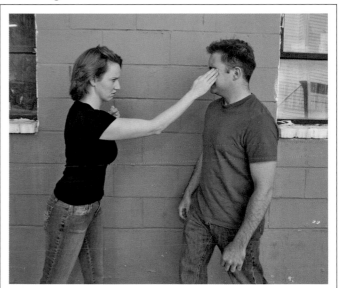

- If a situation clearly has reached the point of imminent danger, don't wait.

- The person who strikes first gains a significant advantage. When that opportunity presents itself, seize it.

- Don't worry that you will be seen as the aggressor.

When it's clear that your safety is in jeopardy, take action.

- It may seem "unfair" or "unsporting" to hit first, but it's an issue of necessity. Consider how unsafe it is to wait for the other person to take initiative.

WHAT IS YOUR GOAL?

Select action that will neutralize the threat

Because so much of a violent attack is outside of our control, we must assume the worst and act quickly. The longer a situation goes unchecked, the more variables we lose control over. Other people may come to the scene, and "x factors" develop beyond our control.

When we realize that physical violence is imminent, we must act. Our action must neutralize the situation, the attack, or the attacker's will (or ability) to continue and in the least

amount of time possible. In low-risk situations, it may be possible to simply defend an initial attack and to make our escape. Many martial arts teach this as the moral high road. However, this can be unrealistic except in the most benign cases. If that strategy happens to work out that way, however, it's a nice bonus for you.

In most situations we should expect to take the "fight" out of our attacker. We should expect to cause tremendous pain

Creating Escape Opportunities

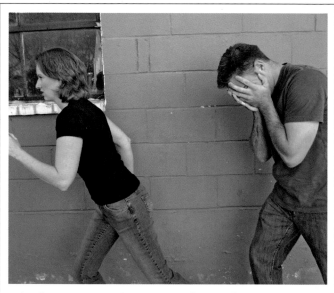

- In a best-case scenario, a quick strike to a vulnerable target will create the time you need to get away.

- When choosing an initial target, look for something sensitive and vulnerable because those targets won't require a perfect direct hit.

- If you strike your assailant and see that he is temporarily incapacitated, you may choose this opportunity to run.

Causing Trauma

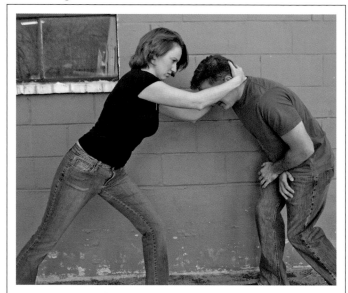

- In some cases the initial strike to a vulnerable target is merely intended to buy enough time for a more effective counterattack.

- A quick strike to the groin can lower someone's defenses in that critical moment when you take the offensive.

- Though the initial shot isn't a "fight ender," use it to buy yourself a head start as you move into more substantial tactics.

or injury (or both). In some cases it might be possible (and slightly more humane) to leave your attacker unconscious. We aim to create sufficient time to allow safe escape for ourselves and anyone else in danger.

Although all this will sound extreme to some ears, let's be clear: Your goal is safety for you and for the people around you. In a later chapter we'll discuss the legal dimensions of this issue. In short: The law defends your right to defend yourself. And from a moral perspective, you have a right to ensure your safety when an unwarranted threat presents itself. Take

the action that is necessary to create safety for yourself and your companions.

Neutralizing the Assault 1

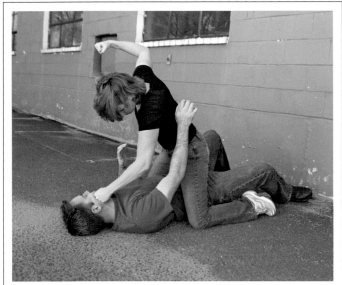

- In many circumstances your assailant will fight back and attempt to continue the assault.

- If escape is impossible or places others in harm's way, it may be necessary to neutralize the attacker by causing severe trauma.

- You're looking for signs that the assailant is no longer interested in continuing the assault. If you're still in danger, then you must continue to fight back.

Neutralizing the Assault 2

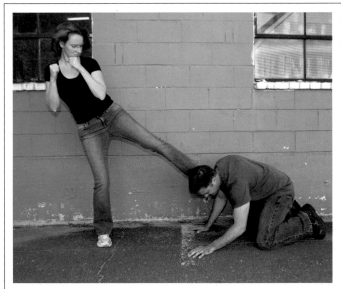

- If you are unable to take the "fight" out of your assailant, it may be necessary to inflict injury or unconsciousness if he continues to pursue you.

- You are looking for the most defensible means of stopping the assailant from

continuing the attack in the most immediate and unquestionable way.

- Although all of this may sound harsh, remember that you may be fighting for your life. You do not know what level of violence this person intends.

THE EYES

A strike to the eyes causes pain and can impair vision

The eyes are a great target for creating intense pain and disturbing someone's vision. They are easily disturbed by even slight contact, and an injury to the eye can persist beyond just the initial contact. Most attacks to the eye target the surface of the eye itself. The cornea is easily damaged and is particularly painful when injured.

Beyond the pain factor, diminishing our attacker's ability to see will make it much easier for us to escape. Taking away our assailant's vision is a great way to create an advantage to strike further or to make our exit.

Another way to attack the eye is to grab the eyelid. Eyelids can be pulled and twisted in a variety of ways that can be tremendously painful.

One benefit to attacking the eye is that the body reacts in predictable ways: The human reflex, when the eye is threatened, is to cover it with the hands. Most people will do this

Eyes Are Sensitive

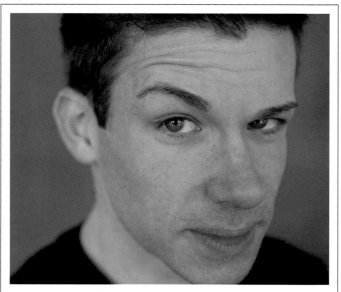

- The primary advantage to targeting the eye is its extreme sensitivity to pain.

- Most people react predictably when the eye is struck: One or both hands cover the eye, vision is severely limited, and pain is immediate.

- When targeting the eye, a direct hit is not necessary. Even moderate contact to the area can disrupt vision and cause extreme discomfort to the eye itself.

Thumbing the Eye

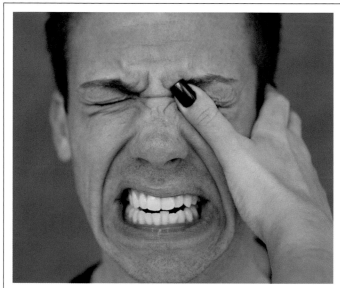

- One of the easiest and strongest tools for targeting the eye is the thumb.

- In close quarters the thumb is often an accessible tool for pressing on the eye.

- You can use the thumb to pull the eyelid closed and then to apply pressure with the pad, tip, or nail.

- When thumbing the eye, anything more than mild pressure can cause serious injury.

instinctively. Although we don't want to depend on this reaction 100 percent of the time, we can predict a good chance of it happening if we make solid contact with the eye. And for many people, even a grazing contact will be enough to provoke that reaction.

Long-range Eye Attacks

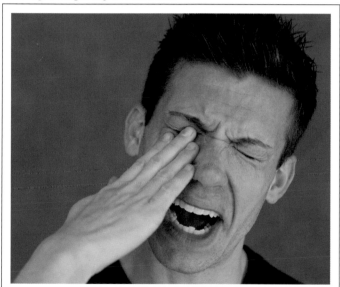

- It is also possible to hit the eye from far away by using the fingers.

- Although the eye is a fairly small target, you can take advantage of a large area of impact because glancing strikes still have an effect.

- Most people lack the training to know how to defend their face from a well-timed strike.

- The ability to hit the eyes from arm's length is a valuable one. It may buy you the time to escape or to move closer and engage stronger tools.

Incidental Eye Contact

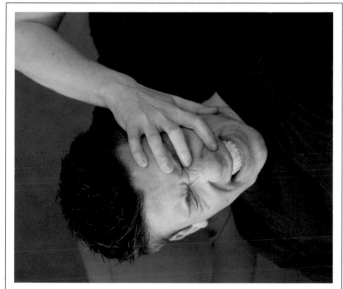

- Sometimes you may traumatize the eye unintentionally. This is in no way a bad thing.

- The eye may be raked, pulled, poked, pressed, rubbed, or otherwise irritated, all to your benefit.

- You may transfer from your hands to the eye materials such as dirt or water. This could happen intentionally or unintentionally.

- Don't forget that many defensive sprays, including pepper spray, are intended to attack the sensitive lining of the eyes.

TARGETS

THE THROAT

Hitting the throat can cause impaired breathing and panic

The throat is another primary target that we should attack to gain the initial advantage.

We can use any hard striking surface of the body to hit the throat, including the hands, fingers, forearms, elbows, head, shin, instep, heel, and knee. In close quarters we can bite the neck to cause intense pain and alarm.

Striking the throat can inflame the trachea (windpipe). The inner lining of the airway can become irritated and swell, causing difficult breathing. Creating difficulty in breathing is a quick way to cause panic and to take an attacker's attention off of you (and onto his own safety).

If we miss the airway, striking either side of the neck alongside the windpipe can sometimes knock people out. The body's mechanisms that regulate blood pressure are housed in the front of the neck, so excess pressure along these structures (from a grab or a quick strike) can sometimes cause

Anatomy of the Neck

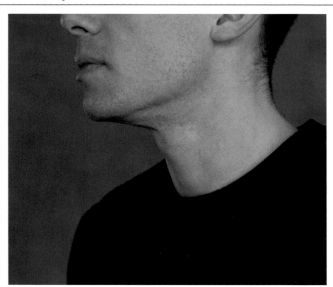

- The windpipe is the most vulnerable area, directly in the center. A strike here, either on or below the voice box, can cause tremendous pain and difficulty in breathing.

- The muscle masses on the side of the neck house the carotid arteries and jugular veins. Some martial arts teach choking techniques in which pressure is applied to the carotid artery to cause unconsciousness.

- Some martial arts also suggest striking the sides of the neck with your hand or forearm, which can sometimes knock someone out.

Attacking the Windpipe

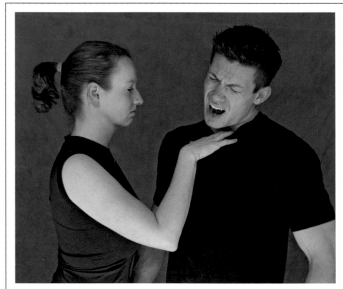

- A strike or press down into the area below the voice box can contact the windpipe directly.

- This causes a quick flash of pain, sometimes accompanied by gagging and panic.

- Traumatizing or injuring the windpipe can create difficulty in breathing, which could be temporary or last for some time.

- This is an area that isn't often touched and as a result remains sensitive.

people to pass out completely. From a humanitarian stand-point, sometimes it's a lot less injurious to an attacker if he just goes unconscious—we will no longer need to cause him any injury in order to escape.

Higher on the Neck

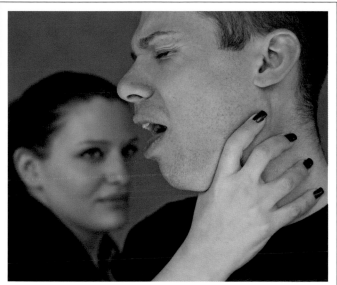

- Other kinds of strikes can attack the voice box itself or above.

- The small bones of the voice box can be injured easily by rough contact or a strike. A direct impact here can be quite painful.

- You can also make contact with the area just above the voice box, beneath the jawline. Pressure on this area causes a feeling of panic and inability to breathe.

- Striking or grasping the throat in these ways causes a reflex response in which the hands come up to try to protect the throat.

Larger Tools

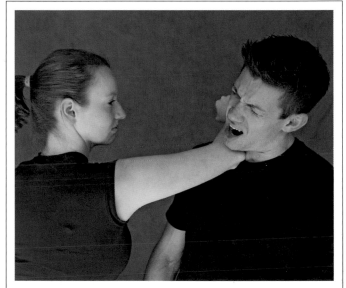

- You can also attack the throat with larger, broader striking surfaces requiring only gross motor movements.

- The forearm and elbow can be delivered to the front, side, or even back of the neck with great effect.

- A punch to the throat or front of the neck delivers a solid impact to delicate areas.

- Situation permitting, a shin, knee, or foot to the throat while wrestling on the ground can be a strong, effective strike.

TARGETS

41

THE GROIN

Attacking the groin causes intense pain and nausea

The groin is one of the primary targets for self-defense because a strike there can be so overwhelmingly successful.

Few men will need an explanation of why the groin is listed here. Even moderate contact can create crippling pain that persists for some time. A strong attack, like a swift kick (to say nothing of seven or eight swift kicks in a row) can often put a man down.

We can target the groin with all kinds of strikes and attacks,

though the easiest are kicks, knees, slaps, and grabs. Grabbing, pulling, and twisting actions can all increase the pain tremendously.

Though often considered comical, injuries to the testicles are quite serious. Many types of testicular injuries require surgical treatment, and some can even be fatal.

When the testicles are struck, the effect on the entire body is similar to the effects of other serious injuries, like a broken

Targeting the Groin

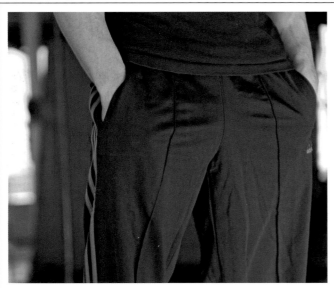

- The groin is an extremely sensitive area, particularly on men.

- Impact to the testicles can be completely incapacitating for a period of several minutes and can even cause life-threatening injury.

- Even a quick or glancing impact can be enough to send a man to the floor.

- Because of the extreme sensitivity, men are likely to flinch or react to any strike in the area of the groin.

Kicking the Groin

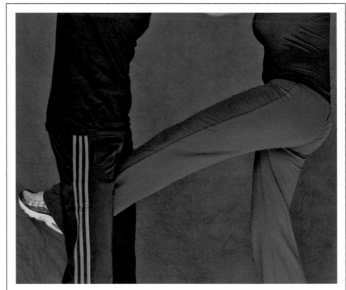

- Kicking the groin can be done from a particularly long distance—farther than most other attacks can be landed.

- It makes little difference what surface is used to deliver the kick; any contact here is devastating.

- Kicks to the groin can be thrown from the front or from behind. They can also be delivered to someone standing behind you.

bone. Often there is some combination of a wave of nausea, inability to stand, dizziness and vertigo, waves of pain that radiate throughout the body, and tingling or loss of sensation in the limbs.

Though the testicles are the most affected target, the rest of the groin is an extremely sensitive area. And sometimes a strike or a kick that lands low on a man's abdomen, at the level of the bladder, will have almost the same effect as a kick to the testicles. The same nerves can be accessed through impact there as well.

The groin is a primary target to strike against a female attacker as well. Although its effect is not as dramatic as the effect on a man, a good kick or strike will cause pain or injury all the same.

Kneeing the Groin

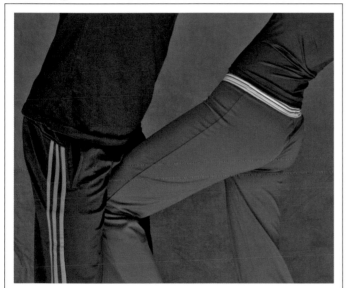

- Perhaps the strongest tool for striking the groin is the knee.

- Broad and solid, the knee is a handy club for attacking. It is powered by the muscles of the core and hips, which are often the strongest in the body.

- A knee that lands anywhere in the vicinity of the groin can have a devastating effect.

- Nine or ten such knee strikes would be even better.

Grabbing the Groin

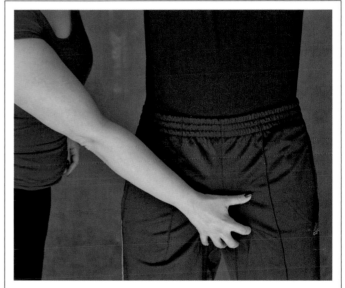

- Not to be overlooked are the various methods of attacking the groin using the upper body.

- The hands have an advantage over the legs when it comes to such attacks because of the ability to grasp, twist, squeeze, and yank.

- All of these actions are tremendously painful and injurious to the testicles.

THE KNEE

Injury to the knee can stop an assailant from pursuing you

The knee joint is the fourth and final primary target. Our purpose when attacking the knee is somewhat different than when attacking the eyes, throat, or groin; here we take away our attacker's ability to chase us.

The knee is most susceptible to impact from the front and the side. Because the joint acts as a hinge, impact on the front can take it beyond its natural range of motion. Damage can be done to the ligaments that control movement and joint integrity, as well as to the patella (the bone that forms the kneecap). A strong impact to the side of the knee is a common sports injury and can often tear the vulnerable anterior cruciate ligament (ACL). Although an ACL injury itself may not stop someone from walking or running, it is often accompanied by other knee injury, such as dislocation or hyperextension. In some cases the ACL injury alone is enough to immobilize the person.

The Knee Joint

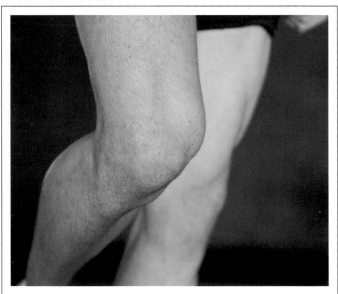

- The knee is held together by a delicate system of ligaments that resists impact from some angles well and from other angles poorly.

- Injury to the knee can make it difficult to walk or run. This means that delivering a knee injury can create tremendously improved opportunity to get away.

- The knee resists damage well from behind and from the inside outward but not from other directions.

Front of the Knee

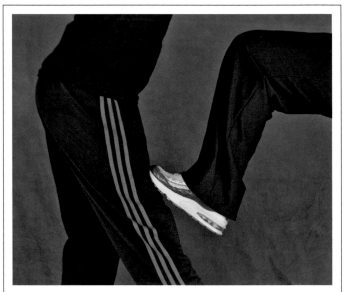

- The front of the knee is a sensitive area.

- A strong strike to the knee can hyperextend it beyond its normal range of motion, causing injury to the tendons and ligaments within.

- Additionally, the kneecap is a sensitive area when struck and is vulnerable to injury. The kneecap can be dislocated or "split" (fractured) with a significant impact.

Some styles of martial arts also practice ways to injure the knee by direct manipulation rather than striking. The most severe and injurious methods involve immobilizing the upper leg, bending the knee, and then rotating the lower leg. These kinds of attacks can easily tear the ligaments that hold the joint together.

Our goal in most crisis situations is to get ourselves away from the danger. What better way to escape an attacker than to remove his ability to follow?

Side of the Knee

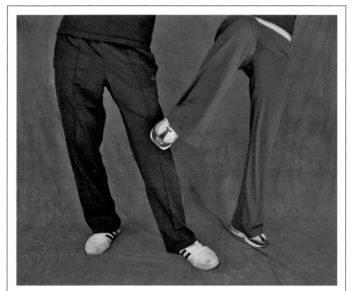

- Impact at the side of the knee can be catastrophic.

- Trauma angled from the outside inward is a common cause of injury to the ACL, one of the ligaments that runs through the knee joint. Injuries of this type to the knee can be quite severe and even permanent.

- These types of injury also make it impossible for someone to run or walk, allowing time and safety for your escape.

Alternate Methods of Attack

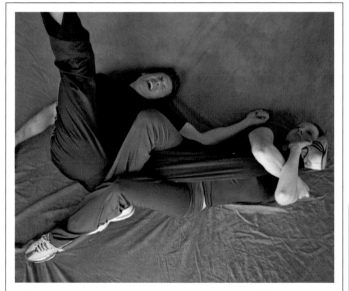

- Some martial arts attack the knee in other ways. The goal is the same: Injury to the knee stops the ability to chase you.

- The kneebar shown here is a method of creating leverage sufficient to break the knee by using several large muscle groups in unison.

- Russian *sambo* is one martial arts system that pioneered methods of attacking the legs.

- The leglocks developed in *sambo* have become popular in other grappling methods and in mixed martial arts.

TARGETS

SECONDARY TARGETS

When the primary areas are unavailable, these are some good alternatives

Although the eyes, throat, groin, and knee are the most effective places to hit because of the dysfunction that striking them causes, several other good options are available. In secondary targets we look for the ability to cause pain and injury that can create distraction.

The list of sensitive areas we can strike is long: nose, temple, cheekbones, back and sides of the neck, ribs, liver (on the right side of the ribcage), kidneys, belly, front and sides of the thigh, shins, ankles, and instep are just a few of the other vulnerable areas we can target.

Although strikes to these areas might not be "fight enders," they can buy us time or help in the damage that we cause.

The Nose

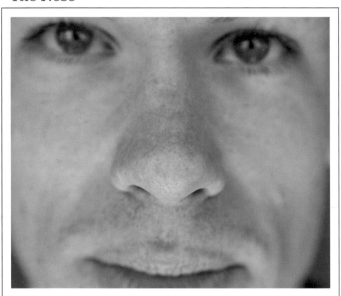

- The nose is a sensitive target that is easy to strike and suffers predictably when hit.

- Besides the pain of impact, trauma to the nose can be momentarily blinding and can cause teary eyes and blurred vision.

- Some impacts will also break the nose, which is likely to bleed and suffer impaired breathing.

The Abdomen

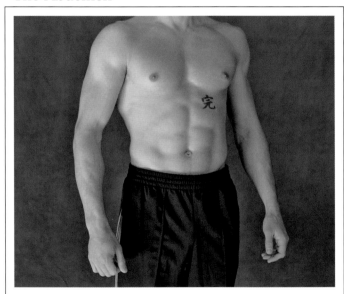

- The abdomen can be a good target for strong attacks, such as a series of knee strikes.

- A hit to the torso can "knock the wind out" of somebody, which causes pain and difficulty in breathing.

- Strong punches or kicks to the side of the torso can also break ribs, which can be immensely painful and sometimes dangerous.

- Because the torso is less sensitive than our primary targets, we typically reserve it for bigger, stronger tools such as knee strikes or a powerful kick.

A stomp on the instep of the foot might not get someone to release a grab, but it might distract him just long enough that we can get our thumb to his eye or our knee to his groin.

Many of these targets can also buy us short periods of time; a strike to the nose sometimes stuns its recipient, as does "knocking the wind out" of someone.

The Thigh

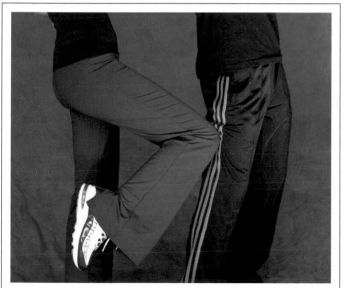

- The thigh is a good noninvasive target that can be struck with great effect but little injury.

- The most effective areas to target are the front and the outside of the thigh. A well-placed knee strike can result in a "dead leg" feeling that can persist for several minutes.

- In close quarters we can also grab, pinch, or rake the tender skin on the inside of the thigh.

The Head

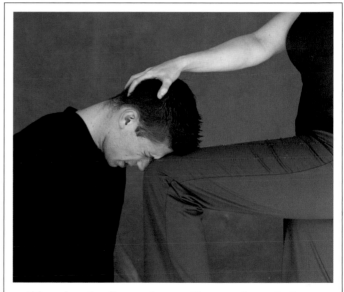

- Although we've discussed the sensitive targets of the eyes, nose, and throat, we can also strike the head as a broader area.

- Bigger tools such as the knee, elbow, and shin can come into play when striking at the entire head.

- You may choose to throw punches at the face, but you should avoid hitting the thick bones of the back of the skull with smaller, more delicate bones such as those in your fist.

TARGETS

STANCE

Place your body in an athletic position in order to take action

Your stance is the most important element of fighting. You want to be in a position that allows you to move, hit, or defend with ease and with power. It should maximize your strength and your body's advantages.

To begin, take a natural step forward with one foot. Most right-handed folks will prefer to keep their right side in back (reverse that for lefties), but that's not always the case. Try standing both ways and see which feels most comfortable.

In this position turn your feet and body to face diagonally forward. Each leg should have a clear path to kick straight ahead, but resist the urge to bow the knees outward—doing so leaves your groin exposed to kicks. Bend your knees and shift your weight into the balls of your feet. Distribute your weight equally between your front and rear legs. We're looking for a balance of mobility and stability.

Tuck your elbows and bring your hands up. You can make

Stance (Front)

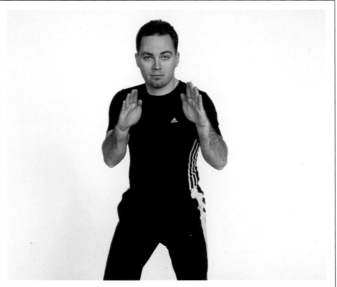

- The ideal stance is an athletic position from which you can move easily in any direction, defend incoming attacks, and throw quick, powerful strikes of any kind.

- The legs are staggered and facing somewhere between diagonal and forward. Each leg has a clear path forward for kicking.

- You present a compact frame and silhouette, which make you a smaller target and harder to hit.

Stance (Side)

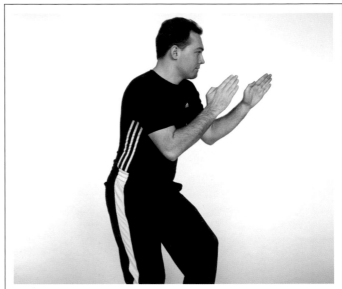

- The ideal width of a stance is a little inside shoulder width; it approximates one natural step forward.

- Most right-handed people prefer to have their right hand in back, but this is not true of everyone. Try both sides and see which feels more natural.

- Be sure to keep your chin down to protect against punches.

- Keep your visual field as clear as possible. Don't block your own line of sight with your hands.

fists with your hands or bring the fingers together if you prefer to have them open. Make sure that you can see down the center, between both hands. Alternatively, you can place your fists on the sides of your face, touching your chin, cheekbones, or eyebrows.

Your Legs

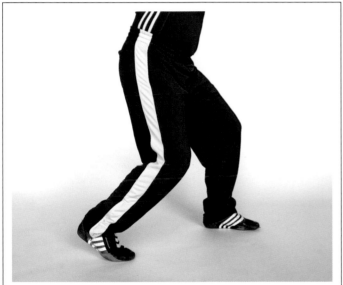

- The knees are bent, which is of the utmost importance for moving well.

- A good knee bend is also critical when it comes to striking with power because it allows you to put your full weight behind your strikes.

- The weight is placed on the balls of both feet and evenly distributed between the right and left.

- The back heel should be raised, allowing you to push forward from your back foot.

Your Arms

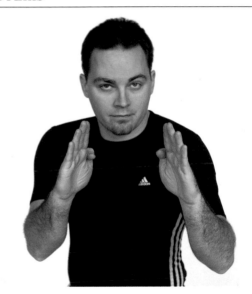

- It's important that the hands are kept up, near the face, where they can be used for defense.

- Keeping the hands up also means they have a shorter route to travel when striking at the eyes and throat.

- Fingers should be kept together for safety.

- The elbows should be tucked in against the body to help with defense both against striking and wrestling-type attacks.

BOXING

THE JAB
The front hand is often the closest tool to your attacker

The most important punch in boxing is the jab. Boxers spend a lifetime perfecting its delivery and use. The jab is a straight punch that travels directly from your stance to its target. It is a quick and snappy punch.

When throwing the jab, we use the front hand—the left hand, for most righties. This hand is one of the quickest tools to reach someone in front of you because it's one of the closest parts of your body to your attacker.

When the jab is thrown, we push off from both legs—especially the back one. Your bellybutton and hips will rotate to face the side, forming a straight line from your punching fist all the way down your arm to your far shoulder.

The jab returns quickly to its starting position by following the same path in reverse. It should take less than a second to hit and return.

It's important to protect yourself as you throw your punch.

Jab—Halfway (Side)

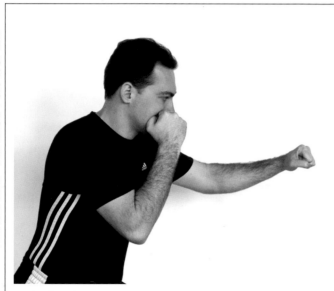

- The first thing that moves when you jab is the fist itself.

- The fist must leave its starting point and head straight for the target without retreating.

- If the hand moves backward first, it will announce the punch before it happens. We call this a "telegraph."

- Avoid telegraphing your punch by focusing on the path straight to the target.

Jab—Full (Side)

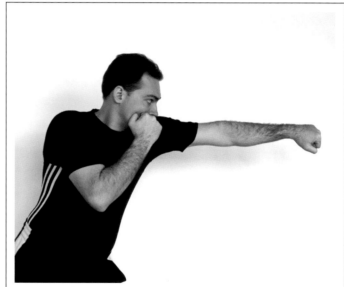

- It's important that you protect your own body when you punch.

- The shoulder is rolled up and squeezed into the cheek to prevent a counterpunch from hitting you in the face.

- The free hand protects the face, and the elbow protects the body.

- Your body has rotated fully to the side on impact. Now it will reverse the process and return to the original stance.

Squeeze your shoulder up against your cheek and tuck your chin down and into your chest. Press your free hand against your opposite cheek to keep your face protected from counterpunches. Also, squeeze your free elbow toward your bellybutton to protect as much of your body as possible from punches and kicks.

Jab—Halfway (Front)

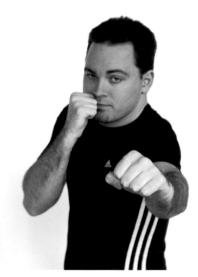

- When throwing the jab, the body turns to push the punch forward. You can see this as the rear shoulder disappears from view in these photos.

- It's important that the elbow does not fly out to the side while the jab is thrown.

- Flaring the elbow weakens the jab and leaves the body unprotected.

- A flared elbow at the start of your jab is also a telegraph. Focus on keeping it in line with your shoulder and fist while you punch.

Jab—Full (Front)

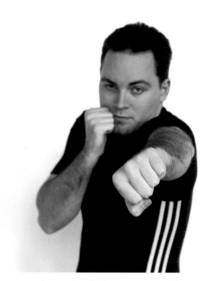

- On impact there should be a straight line from the fist through the front shoulder to the back shoulder.

- The body is pushed from the back foot.

- The fist has turned almost fully thumb-down, and the shoulder is rotated up to protect the face.

- The other hand and elbow are squeezed in to protect you from counterattack.

BOXING

THE CROSS
The rear hand provides a powerful strike when thrown properly

Most people stand with their dominant side behind them because they can throw a powerful cross—a straight punch right down the centerline—with their strongest arm.

Imagine that you're preparing to run a sprint. You bend your knees and crouch down partway, and then, as you hear "go," your legs send you flying from the starting blocks into action.

That same feeling of extending the legs and throwing your body forward is used in almost all athletics, whether you're swinging a baseball bat, a hockey stick, or a golf club, whether you're throwing a football or a baseball or jumping for a basketball. And when we throw the right cross, we'll use that same action again.

As your fist drives forward from its starting point, drive from your back leg. Let the hip and knee come forward as you push—hard—into the ground. Drive the weight of

Cross—Half (Side)

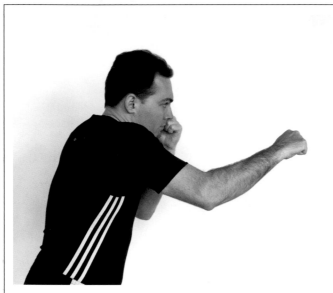

- As with the jab, the hand is the first body part that moves when you throw the cross.

- The fist moves forward to the target without retreating.

- The elbow must stay in line with the shoulder and fist as the punch travels forward rather than flaring out to the side.

- Stand with your dominant side in back, so that you can throw the cross with maximum power.

Cross—Full (Side)

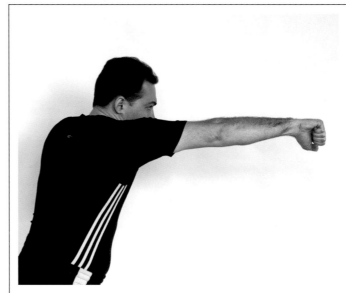

- On impact the chest and hips are turned fully into the punch, driven by the hip, knee, and ankle straightening on the rear side.

- It's important that after impact, the fist returns to its starting point in a straight line rather than looping downward on its way back.

- It's important not to overthrow the cross, which can leave you off balance and undefended. Return to your stance quickly and smoothly in the shortest path possible.

your body into the punch so that it lands with full power. Make sure you begin with both knees generously flexed, so that you can take full advantage of your leg strength as the legs straighten and push you forward.

When the punch reaches full extension (a few inches behind its intended target), pull it back smoothly and quickly down the same path. Be sure it doesn't loop downward or forward, leaving you off balance and undefended.

The three squeezes that we performed with the jab—the shoulder against the face, the fist covering the opposite cheek, and the elbow against the ribs—also apply to the cross. Be sure to protect yourself while you punch!

Cross—Half (Front)

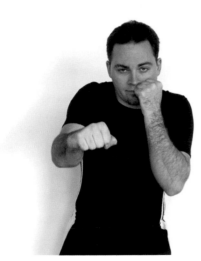

- The cross travels directly down the centerline, straight to its target.

- The rear leg pushes the body forward by extending at the hip, knee, and ankle. This puts the weight of the body into the punch.

- The hips, chest, and shoulders rotate forward into the punch from their original position.

Cross—Full (Front)

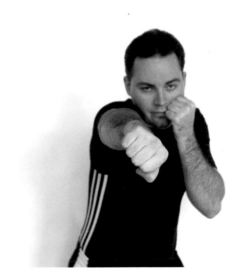

- On impact roll the shoulder up to protect the face while the opposite hand protects the other side.

- Squeeze your free elbow toward the bellybutton to defend strikes to the body.

- The cross can be thrown effectively to the face and to the body. To throw to the body, lower yourself by bending your knees rather than aiming downward.

DEFENSES FOR STRAIGHT PUNCHES

Here are some techniques for defending against the jab and the cross when you're on the receiving end

Straight punches are the most common punches in the boxing range because they take the shortest path to the target (a straight line), and they reach farther than curved punches. When we defend straight punches, we need to make sure we cover up the center alley where these punches are thrown.

Take a second to imagine that someone is standing in front of you. Get into your stance. Imagine the vertical line down the middle of the person's body—if it helps, think of the line of his spine. Now imagine the line down the middle of your body in the same way. Picture the narrow vertical plane that extends between both of these two lines. This is commonly referred to as "centerline."

Covering the Cross

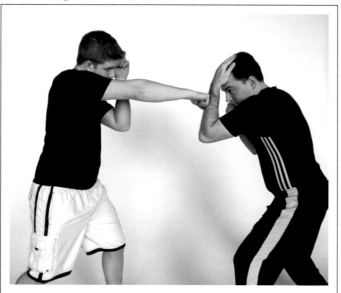

- A "cover" uses your arms to defend against a punch.

- When you cover, the hand is placed on the head, with elbow tucked in and wrist flexed. Impact is absorbed by the arm rather than the head.

- It's important not to have space between your head and your cover, or else you'll punch yourself in the head on impact.

- Covering a punch can be an effective defense even at the last moment.

Slipping the Punch

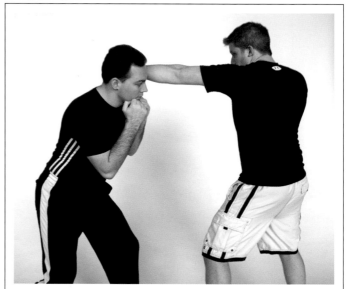

- Slipping, or moving your head off the line of the punch, is one method of defending against punches without your arms.

- Boxers and kickboxers develop good head movement to make it more difficult to strike them effectively.

- When done well, moving the head offline is a safe way to avoid injury. It can be combined with other types of defenses, such as hand defenses or body defenses.

- It's important to stay balanced and mobile while you move your head.

When you throw straight punches, they travel down the centerline, down the alley between your attacker's hands, and typically land on targets that lie on the centerline (the face, the nose, the center of the belly, the groin). It's important that you learn to guard your own centerline to keep those targets protected on your body.

Every martial art or self-defense method has different suggestions for defending against punches. If you decide to do some training, choose a school or gym where you'll test out those defenses in some kind of sparring. Although plenty of things work in theory, you'll want as much hands-on practice as you can find to put these defenses into action.

The key is to develop an "eye" for what someone is about to do—train so that you can accurately predict when someone is about to punch at you and develop the timing to perform your defense so that it is effective. This kind of awareness is critical to defending yourself against punches.

Using "Destructions"

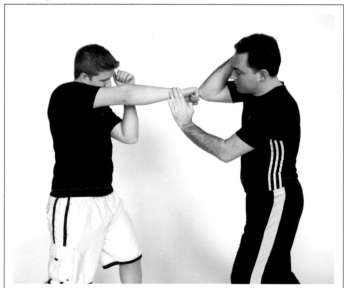

- Destructions are a tactic common to Filipino martial arts, and they involve attacking the incoming arm or leg as a means of defending against a strike.

- Although there is a variety of destructions, one of the most effective ones is to make your opponent strike a harder surface than intended with a weak portion of the hand, arm, or leg.

- Destructions may cause an attacker to punch the tip of the elbow or even the top of the skull, injuring his hand.

Groin Kick Counter

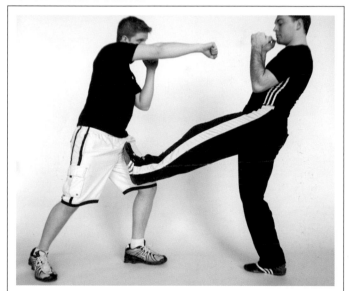

- Many straight punches can be countered with a well-timed kick to the groin.

- Almost all people spread their knees when they punch because it feels natural to step forward while punching.

- Kicking the groin is a good way to take advantage of this opening, causing pain and potentially incapacitating the attacker.

- The groin kick also has the ability to stop the body weight from coming forward into the punch because it can be used to push the hips away.

DEFENSES FOR HAYMAKERS
Untrained attackers are more likely to throw wide, looping punches

The "haymaker" is an untrained punch—a big, looping swing with a lot of oomph behind it. Although it may not be the hallmark of a trained boxer, you don't want to be on the wrong end of one.

The safest defense for any punch is to be too far away. If the attacker can't reach you with the punch, you're safe.

With strikes that have a wide arc, it can also be safe to stand very close to your opponent, inside the arc of the punch. One strategy for getting control of someone who throws lots of haymaker punches is to keep your distance until just after a punch has passed and then to run forward and close the distance between the two of you before the next one comes. Even as the second punch is thrown, you can be safely inside its arc, establishing control and landing strikes of your own.

The higher your awareness level, the earlier you'll see strikes coming. And the earlier you can identify the incoming attack,

Out of Range

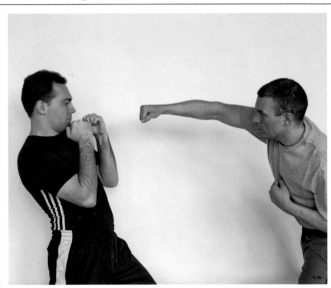

- One of the best defenses against a haymaker-style punch is to be out of range.

- Wide, looping punches can have a lot of power behind them. Avoiding them is a prudent strategy.

- Knowing the right distance to maintain between

  yourself and your attacker is critical.

- Managing that distance is a key skill, born of good awareness and footwork skills.

- Out-of-range defenses can also be paired with a groin kick or other strike.

Covering the Haymaker

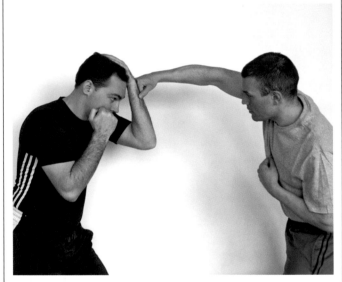

- As with straight punches, you can use a cover to defend against the haymaker.

- By protecting the head with the arm, you protect any delicate, vulnerable areas.

- This defense is more difficult against a haymaker

  because the haymaker develops a lot of momentum by the time it makes impact.

- However, sometimes you are late to defend. The cover provides a valuable defensive option in the last fractions of a second before a punch lands.

the more options (and the better options) you'll have at your disposal. Stopping a haymaker early, before it develops its momentum, is another safe method of defending it.

Intercepting the Haymaker Early

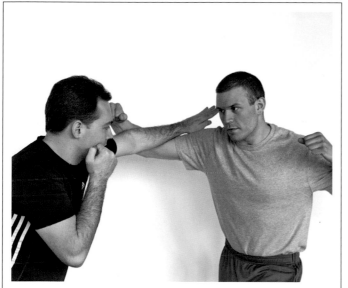

- Early defenses meet less force on impact because they do not wait for the full momentum of the attack to develop.

- The downside to these defenses is that they require a larger deviation from your primary stance and can leave other areas open.

- These defenses require early action and strong commitment to employ. They may also be paired with a counterstrike to improve their effect.

Charging In against Haymakers

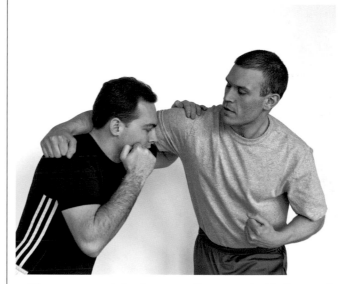

- When you cannot stay far away from the haymaker, sometimes the safest place to go is into close quarters.

- The haymaker relies on distance as its asset and is most dangerous when you stand at arm's length from it.

- By moving inside the arc of the punch, you take yourself out of the place where the haymaker can do the most damage.

- Although moving forward against aggression may be counterintuitive, it can sometimes be one of the safer options.

BOXING

MODIFYING THE BASIC PUNCHES
Alternate striking surfaces give you options for different targets

The basic jab and cross are perfectly fine attacks in themselves, but sometimes we want to adapt them for specific purposes. We can use the same structure and power delivery to throw a variety of strikes, including slaps, palm strikes, eye pokes, elbows, and more.

We can use both the jab and the cross to deliver targeted strikes to the eye. With your palm facing down, hold your fingers straight and together. Throw the punch as you would

otherwise but make contact with the extended fingers to the eye. Aim not only to make impact at the surface of the eye but also to push deeper against it. Throw hard and quickly.

We can also throw the basic punches as open-handed strikes or use the web of the hand between the thumb and index finger. At close range we can use the jab and cross movements to throw elbow strikes.

Another way to adapt the basic punches is to change your

Open-handed Right Cross

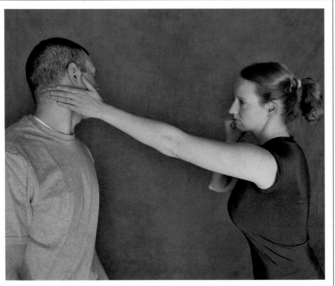

- Some targets aren't ideal for the closed fist. Hard surfaces such as the top of the head can injure the small bones of the hand.

- Punches can be thrown with an open hand, either as a straight punch or in a slapping motion but with

  the same power as a traditional punch.

- Put the body behind your open-handed strikes just as you would with a regular punch. And protect your opposite side as normal.

Jab to the Eye

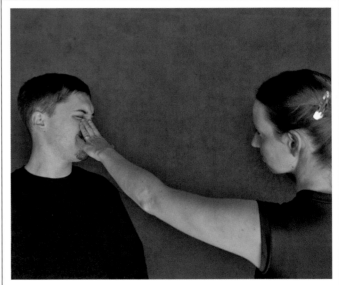

- The same punches can be thrown using the fingers, which add a small amount of extra reach to the strike.

- Because the fingers are not a strong surface, this is limited to soft tissue targets such as the eye, where the fingers will not be injured.

- Sensitive targets such as the eye are ideal because they do not require a heavy impact to create an effective result.

58

level. Bend your knees until the target in front of your shoulders is the midsection or the groin. You can throw powerful punches to the stomach or groin this way without leaving your face exposed to being hit.

Cross with the Web Hand

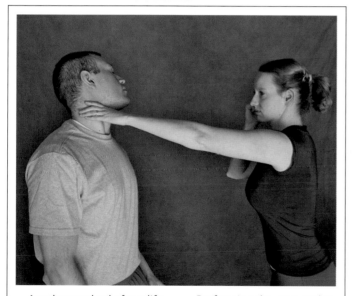

- Another method of modifying the straight punches is to use the web of the hand between the thumb and index finger.

- This strike is often aimed at the throat because of the natural contour of the hand in this position.

- Performing the cross in this way does not diminish the power generated by the body. The turn of the body and participation of the legs are still the same.

Changing Levels and Targets

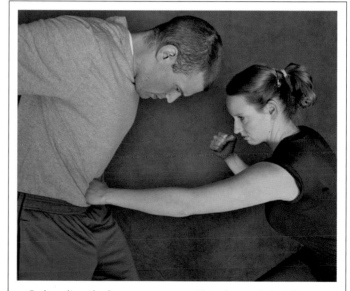

- By bending the knees you can lower the height of your shoulders and, as a result, the height of your punches.

- With a significant level change, you can line up your punches to connect with the abdomen or even the groin.

- This change in height can be difficult to judge on the receiving end, making it a deceptive way to strike.

- Be sure that the change in level is done entirely with the legs and not by slouching with the upper body.

BOXING

59

THE GROIN

The groin is the fundamental target for kicking and kneeing techniques

The groin is a key target because of several considerations: It's easy to reach, it's difficult to defend effectively, it can be struck with any surface, and you don't need to kick above the waistline, leaving your balance substantially unaffected.

It takes very little kicking power to create a massive effect when aiming for the groin, and impact creates a significant (and often predictable) result. There are a number of methods of kicking the groin. Although it's hard to say that any method of kicking the groin is wrong, there are certainly some preferred methods.

One way is to kick straight upward, as though kicking a ball. This is perhaps the easiest and most direct method of bringing

Kneeing the Groin

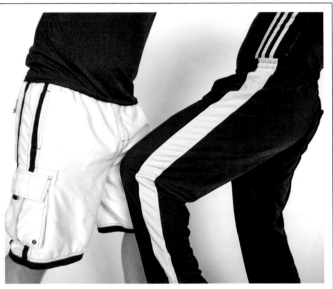

- The knee to the groin is an easy strike to throw with the legs. It has few moving parts and is a simple attack.

- The knee is lifted by some of the strongest muscle groups in the body and is a solid striking tool.

- Kneeing the groin is perfect for close-quarter situations. It requires little room to perform effectively.

- The knee to the groin can also be thrown quite a few times in rapid succession.

Soccer-style Groin Kick

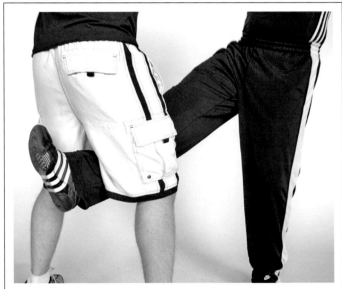

- From longer ranges an easy way to kick the groin is a soccer-style kick that travels upward.

- When kicking this way, the knee is pointed at the target, and then the leg is extended.

- Depending on how far away your target is, you might make contact with your shin, ankle, top of the foot, or toe of your shoe.

- Your footwear is also a determining factor: Shoes with a solid toe make a better striking surface.

the foot to the groin. Contact can be made with the shin, ankle, instep, or toe of the shoe (given appropriate footwear).

Another method is to aim the knee at the target and then snap the foot forward for a quicker style of attack.

Yet another method of kicking the groin is to bring the knee up to the chest and then pump the heel forward, driving into the groin. This method is great for pushing an attacker backward because, in addition to the injury to the groin, it pushes the hips and center of gravity backward forcefully.

Kicks to the groin can be thrown equally well if you are standing behind your assailant. For this purpose, the upward kick is the most suited, but it will connect just as effectively if thrown from the front.

In close quarters the knee is easily thrown to the groin and with the same force and effect as a full kick.

Thrusting Kick 1

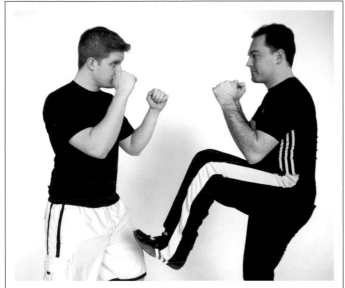

- A thrusting-style kick is a powerful way to attack the groin.

- First the knee is chambered high to the chest.

- From there the leg will push directly forward, as if kicking down a door.

- This kick can target the midsection as well as the groin.

Thrusting Kick 2

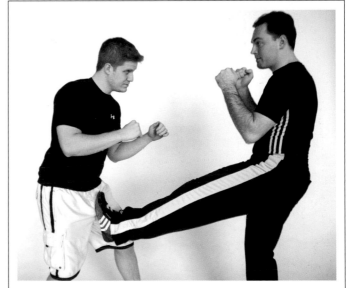

- When the kick is delivered, the force of impact pushes the attacker's hips backward.

- This generates more time (and space) between you and your attacker.

- Lean back with your shoulders and drive your hips forward into the kick.

- Make contact with the heel or the entire sole of the foot.

- This kick requires more distance than the soccer-style groin kick.

LOW LINE KICKS
Other targets below the belt are good low-risk alternatives

In some situations it may be difficult or inappropriate to kick the groin. Instead we may choose from several other low targets for our kicks that are less invasive but equally low risk.

Stomping is a popular and easy way to deliver low line kicks. We can stomp the top of the foot, the ankle, the shin, and the front, side, or back of the knee. In some cases we can even stomp the thigh. Stomps are best delivered with the heel of the foot and doubly so if you are wearing a shoe with

a pointy heel. A focused impact of this kind can do tremendous damage to soft tissue and bony areas alike.

We can kick with the ball of the foot or toe of the shoe to some targets, including the inner and outer thigh and the shins. A good, hard impact on the shin can be extremely painful and even injurious. Likewise, a kick that hits the thigh about halfway between the hip and knee, on either the inside or outside pants seam, can cause a "dead leg" sensation. These

Stomping the Foot

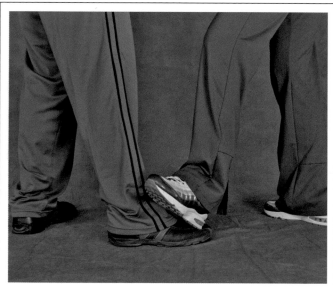

- One strike that is simple to deliver is a stomp to the top of the foot.

- This is delivered with the heel, striking to the more delicate bones on the instep (top) of the foot.

- A stomp can also be done to the shin, depending on position.

- Stilettos or other pointy-heeled shoes can increase the damage done by a well-placed stomp.

Kicking the Shins

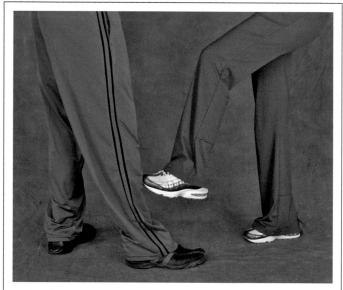

- The shins are a sensitive target and are easy to reach with kicks and stomps.

- A solid strike to the shins can impair walking for a short period of time.

- Kicks to the shins are enhanced by footwear. They can be thrown with the toe or the bottom of the shoe.

- If the attacker is behind you, a kick to the shins can be delivered backward with the heel.

areas are tender and unaccustomed to impact. The thigh can also be struck by using the knee or by swinging our shin like a baseball bat.

Striking the Thigh

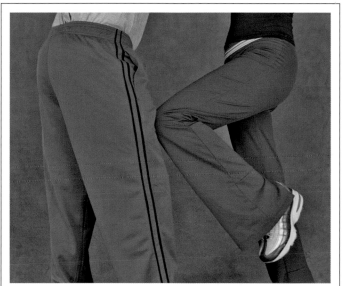

- The thigh can be struck solidly with the knee from the front or side.

- The strike is similar to the knee to the groin but less invasive.

- Another common way to attack the thigh is to kick using the shin, swinging the leg like a baseball bat, or to kick with the shoe from farther away.

- The outside of the thigh is particularly sensitive to impact and creates the "dead leg" feeling when struck.

Stomping the Knee

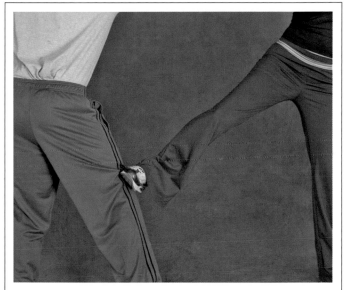

- A stomp to the knee is a strong attack that can cause tremendous injury if the knee is bent in an unnatural direction.

- Stomps to the front of the knee can hyperextend the joint and cause difficulty in walking.

- Stomping the side of the knee is potentially the most injurious.

- The stomp to the knee can be done from a long distance, taking advantage of the length of the leg.

THE HEAD: STANDING
Kicking the head while standing can be a high-risk maneuver

A number of martial arts teach and encourage kicking to the head. Although this can be an effective maneuver for highly trained individuals, it should be considered "high risk" and not used carelessly.

The major risk of kicking high is that your balance is compromised. Standing on one foot is not the stance for a wrestling match because it will end with you on the ground and quickly. Even if your attacker doesn't manage to catch your kick, a solid impact can throw you off balance, and you may wind up on the ground anyway.

Additionally, the power needed to deliver a strong head kick is significant. If you can throw well at head height, you can definitely throw a powerful kick to low areas.

As a rule, keep kicks at the waistline or below. Doing so dramatically reduces the risk of having someone grab your leg while you're kicking, and that means greater safety for you.

Kicks to the Head 1

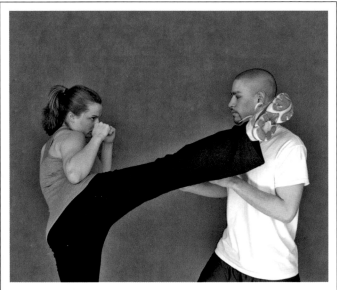

- Many martial arts teach and advocate the development of kicks to the head.

- A kick to the head can be a powerful strike, given the amount of power that kicks can generate.

- Kicks to the head can be thrown with the shin, instep, heel, sole, ball of the foot, or toe of the shoe.

- In sports such as kickboxing and mixed martial arts, a kick that lands solidly on the head often scores a knockout.

Kicks to the Head 2

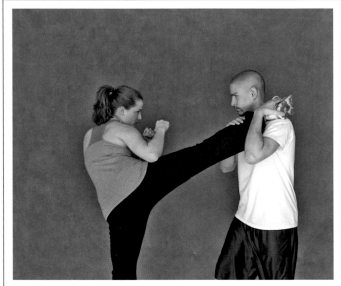

- On the other hand, kicking high above the waist is also a high-risk maneuver.

- To bring one's own leg that high can compromise balance, especially upon impact.

- The greatest danger is that your opponent will be able to grab your leg—or the rest of your body.

- It is extremely difficult to stop someone from taking you to the ground in this position, and the danger of falling on your head is significant.

The exception to this rule is this: If you can bring the head down to the waistline, it's a good target. In this case you'll almost always throw knees instead of full kicks. But it's a great way to bring your leg and your attacker's head together!

Bringing the Head Down

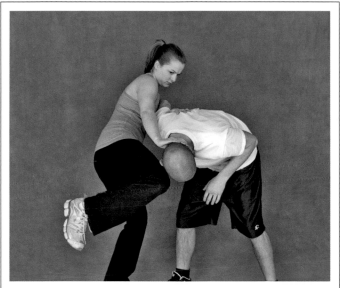

- Sometimes you can bring the head down to waist level. This is a much better option for kicking or kneeing the head.

- Holding the head at waist level makes it difficult for an opponent to move or strike effectively.

- Be sure to keep your legs safely away, so they cannot be grabbed.

- In a position such as this, nine or ten quick, hard knee strikes to the head can be a solid strategy for trying to end a fight.

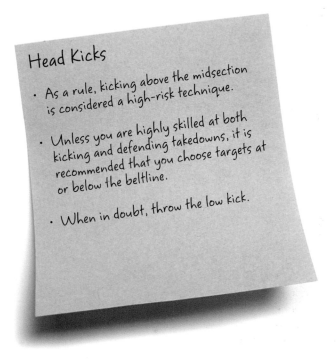

Head Kicks

- As a rule, kicking above the midsection is considered a high-risk technique.

- Unless you are highly skilled at both kicking and defending takedowns, it is recommended that you choose targets at or below the beltline.

- When in doubt, throw the low kick.

THE HEAD: DOWN
Targeting the head is much lower risk when it's closer to the ground

Kicking the head has its risks when you're standing, but if your attacker's head is on the ground, it's a whole different story. Much of the risk is diminished if your kick is aimed below your own waistline. This makes kicking or kneeing the head a much more attractive option.

When trying to get away from someone, you may be able to knock him to the ground, but this doesn't mean that the danger is over. This may be only a momentary reprieve before the assault resumes. Kicking the head while your attacker is down (or nearly down) can be an effective tactic in this situation.

If your attacker tries to grab at your legs, choose your opportunity carefully. Control one or both of his arms if you can. Deliver a knee to the face, the side of the head, under the jaw, or anywhere else along the head and neck that you can.

Against Takedowns

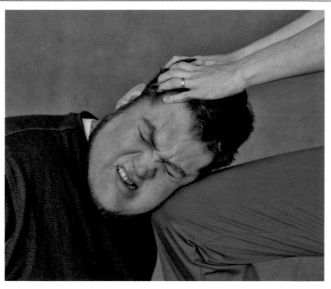

- Some attackers will try to drag you to the ground by the legs. This can be an opportunity, if done carefully, for you to knee the head.

- Although untrained attackers may try to grab you like this, wrestlers are also trained to lower their body and grab legs in this way.

- The most available target for a knee here is the head. It's a strong strike and a defenseless target in this position.

- Control your attacker with your hands or forearms to be sure you aren't grabbed.

Soccer-style Kicking

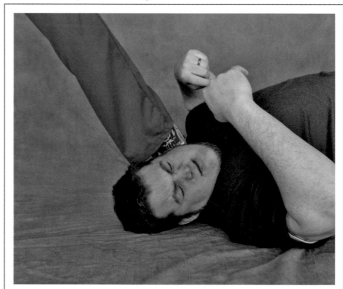

- When an attacker is down, there are opportunities to throw very powerful kicks.

- In this position you can deliver kicks to the head as well as to the neck, collarbone, ribcage, groin, and thighs.

- The primary danger, when kicking an opponent who is down but still fighting, is that your leg may be grabbed.

- Choose your opening and then throw the kicks with everything you have.

If he's closer to the ground, you can deliver a great variety of kicks and stomps. These can be aimed not only to the head but also to the midsection (especially the ribs) or to the groin, knees, and ankles. Assess your footwear and the available targets and then go to work.

GREEN ● LIGHT

Part of fighting back effectively is the readiness to take advantage of any opportunity in order to turn the fight in your favor. If that means kicking someone in the head as he tries to get off the ground, so be it. The old adage "Never kick a man when he's down" really doesn't apply to self-defense. In our field, it's encouraged.

Stomping

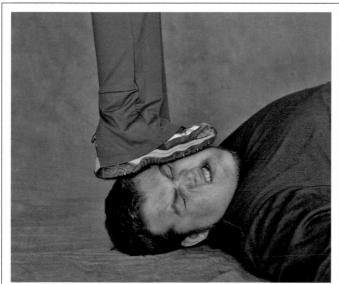

- The stomp is another strong technique that is readily available when your attacker is down.

- Stomp with the heel of your foot rather than the whole sole.

- If your shoes have a pointy heel, the damage from the stomps is greatly increased.

- Almost any target can be appropriate for a stomp, although primary ones include the head, groin, neck, ribs, knees, ankles, and hands.

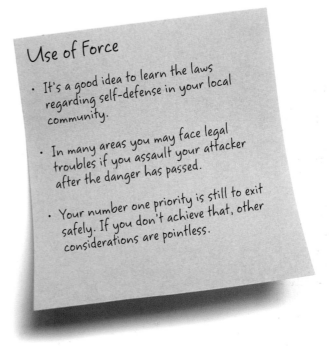

Use of Force

- It's a good idea to learn the laws regarding self-defense in your local community.

- In many areas you may face legal troubles if you assault your attacker after the danger has passed.

- Your number one priority is still to exit safely. If you don't achieve that, other considerations are pointless.

THE BODY

Striking the body effectively requires knowing when it's appropriate and when it's not

Kicking and kneeing the body are a funny middle ground between delivering low line kicks and head kicks. Although they aren't quite as risky as kicking up high, they can still carry risk. The most important thing is to know *when it's appropriate to attack the body*.

The biggest risk when striking the body with your foot, leg, or knee is that this is when it's easiest for someone to grab it. A wrestling match while standing on one leg will end badly for you.

The best bet, if we plan to kick or knee the body, is to use what's called an "underhook." This is a method of controlling the shoulder that we'll discuss at length in the next chapter.

Caught on One Leg

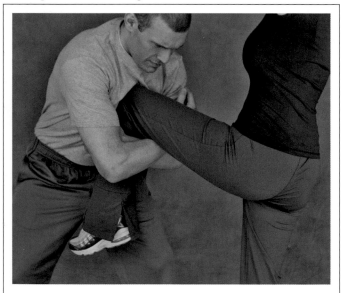

- When kicking or kneeing the body, the primary risk is that your leg will be grabbed.

- Wrestling while standing on one leg is not a winning proposition. It's a dangerous position that should be avoided at all costs.

- Without both legs on the ground, it's hard for you to maintain balance or to throw any strike with power.

- It's also nearly impossible to avoid going to the ground, which is *not* the place you want to be.

Straight Knee

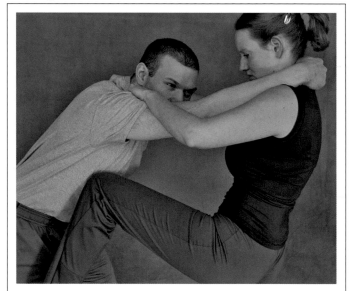

- When you are able to control one of your attacker's arms, this can be a safe time to throw the knee to the body.

- By controlling the arm, you keep it clear of your leg while you strike. Although this strike would be risky otherwise, the upper body position makes it much less so.

- Sometimes this method of control on the upper body stretches the torso, making the ribs more susceptible to injury and the knee strike even more effective.

The underhook is a means of keeping the attacker's arm too high to grab your leg—meaning that, with an underhook established, you can feel free to whale away at the body with knee strikes.

Although the ribcage isn't quite as desirable a target as our primary ones, several strong knee strikes can do a lot of damage. At the very least, they can knock the wind out of your attacker. Sometimes strikes thrown to the right side of the body will injure the liver, which can incapacitate someone for a period of time.

As with all the striking methods we've discussed, plan to throw several strikes in a row with a vicious level of speed and power. If you can establish a strong underhook and plan to knee the body, fire away as many as you can until the situation changes, meaning either that you lose your underhook or that he falls down. If the strikes don't have the desired effect, change to another target.

Kneeing the Side

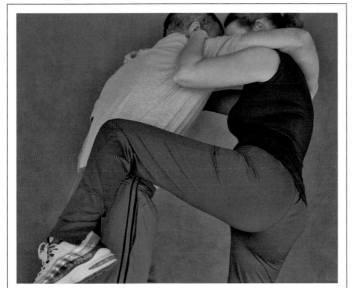

- With the arm controlled, you can also safely throw a knee to the side of the body.

- Knees to the sides can be thrown in a straight line while standing off to the side, or they can be delivered on an arc.

- Knees to the sides of the body can target the ribcage and can cause considerable damage.

- Some methods of throwing the knee target the liver on the right side of the torso. This can be a devastating strike.

Kicking the Body

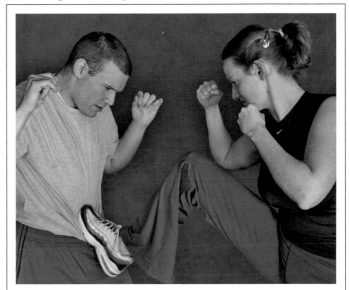

- Kicks to the body are slightly lower priority than kicks to the groin and other low targets, but they are still an effective technique.

- One powerful method of kicking the body is to raise the knee and drive the heel forward, with a thrusting action. This kick can target almost anywhere on the torso with good effect.

- Kicks to the body can be thrown from farther away than the knees and are one of the longest-range attacks you can launch.

FROM BEHIND
Kicks are one of the best striking options when you are surprised from behind

It can be difficult to throw strikes with your hands when caught from behind, but kicking is another story. The legs are extremely powerful when thrown backward, and these types of kicks are useful at a variety of angles.

The biggest priority when grabbed from behind is to act quickly. Waiting allows a bad situation to become worse. If you find yourself surprised from behind, you can deliver a sharp kick backward with the heel of the foot. Remember that you won't be able to see where you're kicking, so you'll need to find your targets by feel (and a little bit of intuition). You might throw your heel backward at the knee and shin or downward onto the top of the foot—which might be visible.

Foot Stomp from Behind

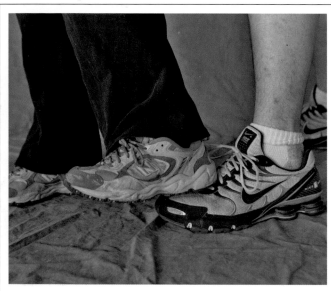

- Foot stomps are one of the easiest strikes to throw against someone who surprises you from behind.

- Drive your heel down onto the top of the foot, targeting the sensitive instep.

- The foot stomp shouldn't be used as a sole strategy but can create a momentary distraction that allows you to switch to more severe tactics.

Heel Kick to Groin

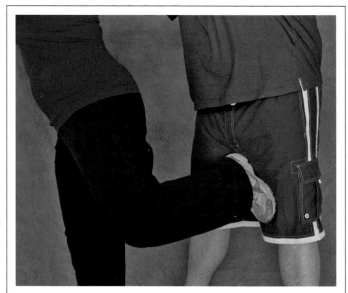

- Another kick you can throw when attacked from behind is the heel kick to the groin.

- Raise your heel quickly behind you, driving your foot into your assailant's groin.

- The heel kick is a quick action that can easily catch someone by surprise.

- This kick is deceptively powerful because it's delivered by strong muscles.

In very close quarters, throwing a stomp might be difficult, but unless the attacker is much taller than you, you can raise your heel up to strike the groin. Although it's not a particularly powerful strike (especially compared with stomps), an impact at the groin can be effective.

If you're lifted off the ground from behind, a kick backward is a terrific idea. Pump your foot backward and see if you can connect with your assailant's groin or knees. You can even kick backward with both feet, provided you stay prepared to catch yourself if he lets go. You'll want to keep your feet

underneath you in case you need to catch your balance suddenly (and you will, especially if you connect solidly with the groin). Be prepared to stop your fall if released—you don't want to make a bad situation worse by knocking him down—on top of you.

Backward Stomp to Knee

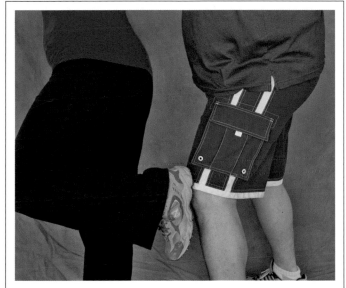

- Another target when you are surprised from behind is the knee.

- In order to deliver this kick, bring your knee forward, aim your heel at the knee behind you, and drive the foot backward.

- The trickiest part of targeting the knee in this position is that you cannot see it—you must do this stomp entirely by feeling where your attacker's body is.

Groin Kick When Lifted

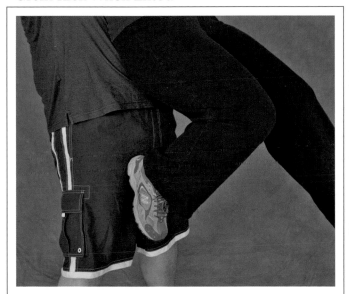

- If you are lifted off the ground, you can still deliver a heel kick to the groin.

- You can actually kick backward with both feet, alternating quickly and repeatedly.

- In this position accuracy is quite difficult, so multiple

kicks are favored because it improves your odds of landing a successful kick.

- Make the actions short and quick. If you are dropped by your assailant, it will be easier to land on your feet if they stay mostly underneath you.

INTRODUCTION TO THE CLINCH
Take control of an attacker who tries to wrestle with you

Martial artists have divided combat into a number of areas, often categorized into "ranges" or "phases" of fighting. Different arts or styles might focus on one or two ranges or phases. Here we'll divide combat into four ranges for the purposes of this book: kickboxing, trapping, clinch, and the ground.

It's essential that we begin our training by learning functional tools in each of these ranges and putting them to use in a variety of training methods. Different arts approach each range with a unique approach or skill set, so there are many options out there. Some folks might focus on one or two ranges, whereas other folks might want to reach a higher level of proficiency in all of them.

In addition to the four basic ranges, we need to consider the presence of weapons, multiple attackers, situational concerns (such as bystanders in jeopardy), environmental concerns (such as fire, stairs, or traffic), and other miscellaneous

Kickboxing Range

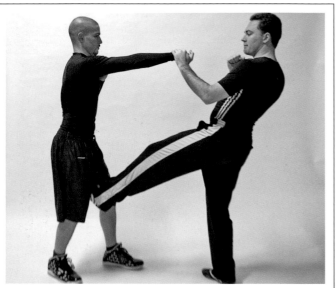

- The boxing/kickboxing range is a distance from which punches and kicks are thrown.

- The kickboxing range is the longest distance in unarmed combat.

- The most important skills in this range are stance and footwork because they dictate your ability to offend and defend whenever necessary.

- Many martial arts, including karate, kung fu, tae kwon do, and kickboxing, practice this distance of fighting.

Trapping Range

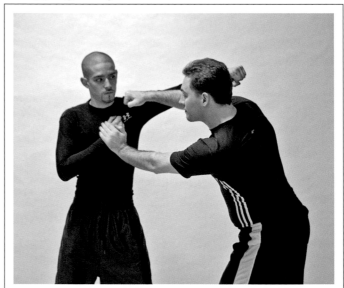

- "Trapping" is a set of techniques that briefly immobilizes or holds an attacker's arms or legs.

- The primary purpose of trapping is to clear a path in order to hit successfully.

- If an attacker puts his hands up to block a punch, you can temporarily trap the hand in order to land a punch.

- The trapping range is the next-closest distance after the boxing/kickboxing range.

issues (such as the presence of graspable clothing).

To be complete, our training should allow us to experience each of these ranges, mixed with each of the above concerns. Through this we will come to familiarize ourselves with—and know from experience—the options that best suit each of us individually.

ZOOM

Statistically the most common attacks a man faces are (1) a big haymaker and (2) an attempted tackle. Women are more likely to be attacked by (1) being approached from behind, grabbed, and dragged to the ground or (2) being approached from the front, grabbed, and dragged to the ground. Because of this, the clinch range is an essential part of training for both genders.

Clinch Range

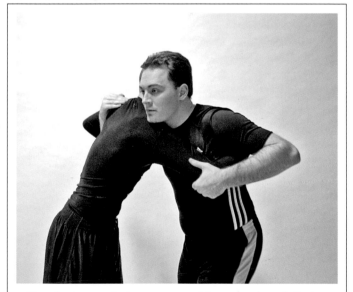

- The clinch range is the closest possible distance between two people while standing.

- In the clinch your goal is to control your attacker by manipulating his body. This may include techniques from wrestling, judo, *sambo*, and other grappling styles.

- A large portion of clinch training involves delivering takedowns and throws and learning to defend them.

- The clinch range also lends itself to close-range striking of all kinds, including punches, kicks, elbows, headbutts, and knees.

The Ground

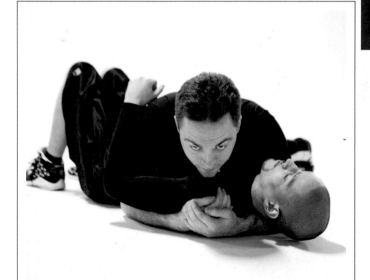

- Some types of assaults may involve wrestling on the ground.

- Several martial arts—most notably Brazilian Jiu-Jitsu, judo, and wrestling—spend a significant portion of their training time on ground fighting.

- Fighting on the ground typically includes controlling your opponent (or escaping his control).

- Ground-fighting training may also include "submission" techniques, which are methods of disabling by choking him unconscious or breaking his arm or leg.

WRIST CONTROL
The wrist is the first handle you use to control your opponent's body

The first of our four fundamental handles of control is perhaps the most difficult. The wrist, because it is so far from the center of the body and center of gravity, can be tricky to use in order to gain control. However, it presents itself because it is often the first handle within our reach.

It is nearly impossible to engage someone physically without presenting your wrist within his arm's reach. We can gain control of the wrist by grasping it and pushing it into the bellybutton, toward the center of gravity. Pushing, in the clinch range, is entirely driven by the lower body. We place one foot behind us for support, and we drive our hips forward, pressing our center of gravity into our attacker.

If you are fighting for control, and you find yourself deadlocked against someone who pushes back, move to one side or the other and push forward from a new angle. This change makes it difficult for the opponent to establish his balance

Controlling the Wrists

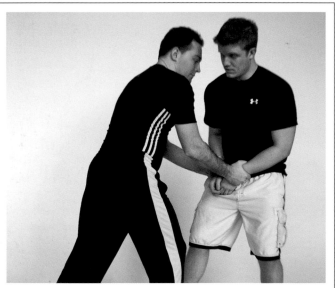

- When controlling the wrists, the primary goal is to affect the center of gravity.

- Capture one or both of your attacker's wrists and push them into the center of the body.

- Drive one side of your body forward, so that you can push your weight into him.

- The power of the drive forward comes from the rear leg. Place it in line directly behind you as you push forward into your attacker.

Grip: Thumb Up

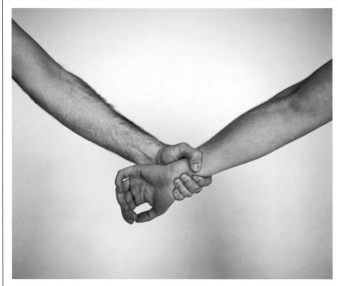

- The most common way people grip the wrist is with the thumb on top.

- The wrist can be grabbed with the same-side hand (right against left) or with the opposite one (right against right) with equal effect.

- The weakest point in the grip is where the thumb lies. If your wrist is grabbed, twist out against the thumb.

against you. Avoiding deadlock is a good way to conserve your energy and use it more efficiently so that your assailant tires more quickly than you do.

•••••••••••••• GREEN ● LIGHT ••••••••••••••

The wrist can be a good handle to grab when you first enter into the clinch range. You may use it as a transition into a more substantial handle because it will provide you momentary safety from punches or grabs as you do so. Experiment with different grips and see which ones transition most comfortably to your other clinch controls.

Grip: Thumb Down

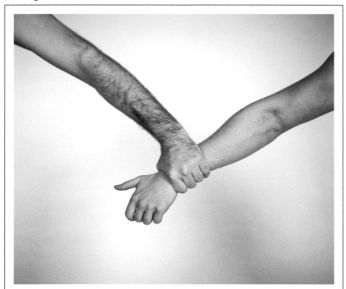

- Some people prefer to grab with their thumb down.

- This is another effective way to grasp the wrist and can be done using either hand.

- The different grips do not have inherent advantages over each other but require

different methods of escape.

- Twisting out against the thumb is still the strongest method of breaking the grip, but with the thumb-down grip, you must twist in the opposite direction of the thumb-up grip.

Two Hands against One

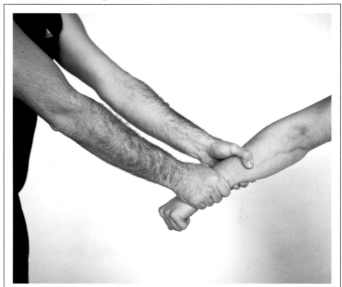

- One strong way to control a wrist is to grasp it with both hands.

- This can be done with both thumbs up, like holding a baseball bat, or with the thumbs together, like holding the top of a steering wheel.

- Although two hands to one (sometimes abbreviated "2-on-1") is a strong grip, the disadvantage is that both of your hands are busy, whereas your opponent has one hand free.

BICEP CONTROL

Controlling the bicep is important for moving an attacker and limiting his ability to strike you

Controlling the bottom of the bicep at the crook of the elbow is a strong way to gain control of your attacker's upper body. Engaging at the bicep can grant you safety from strikes and from more dangerous grabs and chokes.

At the bicep we first experience the importance of "inside position," meaning we want our attacker's forearms outside

our own. If we can dominate the middle position, we have much more control over our movement and balance.

Establishing control over the biceps makes it difficult for an attacker to hit us, which is a tremendous boon at this close distance. Grabs and chokes are also difficult to establish if we maintain inside position. In fact, the more experienced you

KNACK SELF-DEFENSE FOR WOMEN

Controlling the Biceps

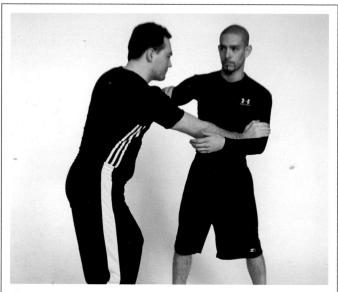

- When you control the biceps, you continue to drive one side of your body forward, pushing into the attacker's center of gravity.

- The bicep control is a bit stronger than wrist control and is an easier place to maintain contact.

- It's important to tuck your elbows against your sides when controlling at the biceps—this increases the strength of your position tremendously.

Inside Position

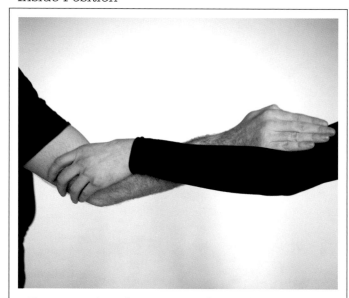

- The person whose forearms are on the inside has an advantage over the person whose forearms are on the outside.

- With the inside position, you can better control your opponent. You can prevent him from striking or grabbing at you.

- When you have the inside position, it is also much tougher for your opponent to prevent you from striking him.

- If you find your arms on the outside, swim them underneath your opponent's forearms and take the inside position.

become with controlling the biceps, the harder it is for anyone to grab you from the front, including chokes.

As with wrist control, it's important to push yourself forward from your rear foot, driving one side of your body into your attacker's center of gravity. Be careful not to overcommit your weight and take yourself off balance. Keep your head up and your shoulders over your hips to avoid taking a fall or an accidental headbutt.

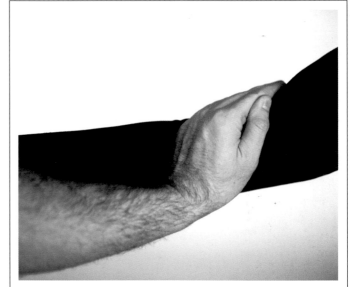

•••••••••••••• GREEN ● LIGHT ••••••••••••••

Controlling the biceps is a simple and powerful way to take the advantage. Practice this method of control as much as possible. Try to continue walking forward the entire time, braced by your rear foot. By applying continuous pressure, you can keep your attacker off balance and make it difficult for him to establish control over you.

Bicep Grip 1

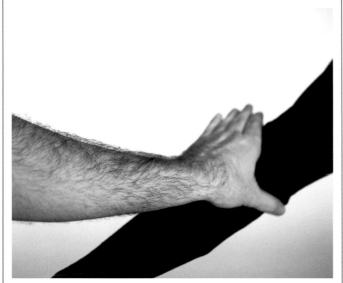

- The first appropriate grip for the bicep uses the web of the hand between the thumb and index finger.

- Grip at the bottom of the bicep in the crook of the elbow.

- If the thumb is extended sideways from your own forearm, it can be injured. Be careful when using this grip to keep the thumb in line with the forearm.

- This grip has a long reach.

Bicep Grip 2

- The second grip for bicep control uses the bottom corner of your palm.

- Place the pinky side of your hand into the crook of the elbow. Cup the outside of the arm with your fingers.

- When using this grip, keep your thumb tucked tightly against the side of your hand.

- Although this grip doesn't reach quite as far as the first one, it is a stronger position and removes the risk of injury to the thumb.

SHOULDER CONTROL: UNDERHOOK

Elevating the elbows takes away your attacker's ability to drag you to the ground

As we continue moving inward toward the center of the body, our third handle for control is the shoulder. We control it using a technique called an "underhook."

To establish an underhook, stand face to face. Reach under your opponent's shoulder and cup your hand over the top from behind. Pull it strongly to you. At the same time lift your elbow to the side to bring his elbow away from his ribcage. As you pull on the arm, rotate it so that his hand points to the ground and his elbow sticks up.

After you have your underhook established, pull as hard as you can! The harder you pull the shoulder to you, the more difficult it will be for your opponent to free his arm.

The Underhook

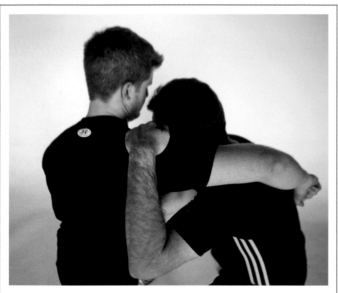

- Controlling the shoulder is done by moving the elbow away from the body and rotating the hand downward.

- With a single arm in the underhook position, cup over the shoulder and hug it to your body.

- Pull strongly in this position, so that the opponent cannot escape your control.

- With only one underhook, you want to place your foot in front of your opponent's. This position makes it difficult for him to drag you into a headlock.

Double Underhooks

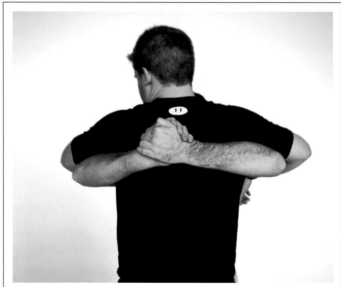

- When possible, it is advantageous to have underhooks on both sides of the body.

- Depending on the size of your opponent, you may be able to join your hands together behind his back.

- If you can't reach, cup each shoulder individually or grasp the back of the shirt with both hands.

- Be sure to elevate his elbows away from his body.

The primary advantage of the underhook is that it prevents an assailant from grabbing around your body or around your legs. By establishing underhooks, you keep his arms above yours. This is no small advantage; it can mean the difference between standing and fighting or being dragged to the ground by a bigger, heavier attacker.

Underhooks are a primary tool used in freestyle and Greco-Roman wrestling. Although they are used in other martial arts, their primary development has come from the Western wrestling tradition.

Prevent Takedowns

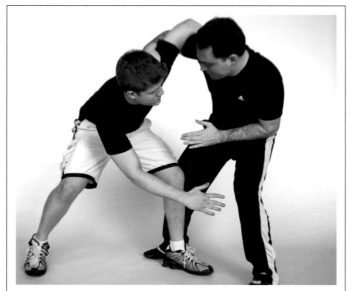

- One of the key strengths of the underhook is its ability to prevent someone from grabbing around your body or legs.

- By having your arm underneath your attacker's and establishing a strong underhook, you deny him access to your torso and lower body.

- If you lose the underhook, swing your arms back inside and underneath to re-establish it.

- Keeping the underhook is essential to good takedown defense.

Underhook and Head Control

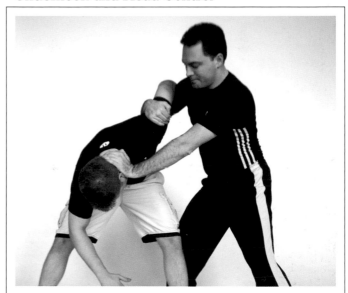

- With a single underhook, one way to improve control is to push the head down and away with the free hand.

- Maintain a strong pull on the shoulder and an equally strong push on the head to keep your attacker restrained.

- This is a strong method of controlling the upper body and is ideal for leading a noncompliant subject.

- In this position you can throw strikes with your knee to the thigh, midsection, or head.

NECK TIE

The neck is a powerful handle for controlling the body and balance

Establishing control at the neck is a strong way to manipulate the body and balance. By directly moving your attacker's spine around, you can push and pull him out of balance and into your strikes.

With the neck tie, we seek the inside position, as we did with bicep control (and the "underneath" position of the underhook). This allows us better control and reduces some of the risk of being hit by your opponent while your arms are busy controlling the neck. After we have a neck tie established, we can strike with the free hand, using punches, elbows, or the thumb to the eye. Or if you prefer more control, you can use both arms to establish a "double" neck tie, with both hands on the neck and both forearms against the chest. This is a particularly strong position for pulling and pushing your attacker off balance and striking with your knees.

It's important to remember that with all clinch handles, we

Double Neck Tie

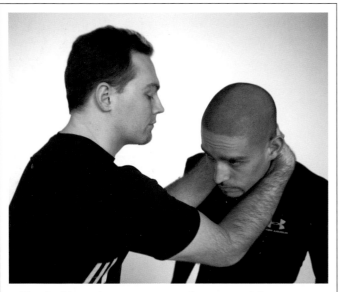

- The double neck tie controls the head and neck strongly and is excellent for moving someone around.

- Maintain a strong push forward with the elbows against the chest while pulling continuously with both hands.

- Squeeze your forearms together underneath the jawbone to make it difficult for your attacker to pull away.

- This position is extremely hard to escape when strongly established.

Preventing Grabs and Takedowns

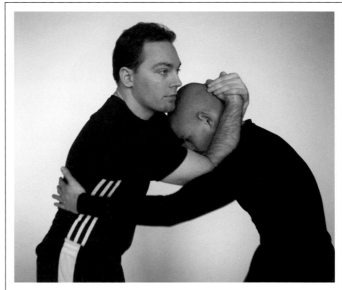

- One key role of the double neck tie is the forward pressure of the forearms.

- The lower third of the forearm, closest to the elbow, acts as a barrier when someone attempts to grab you.

- By pushing against the chest or collarbones, you guarantee yourself distance between the two of you—the distance of your upper arm.

- This creates a strong frame that makes it difficult for an attacker to grab you around the torso or legs.

must continue driving our opponent off balance. Because his arms are free, standing still invites him to hit or grab at our midsection and lower body. Yank him around to keep him off balance and unable to hit you successfully.

Double Neck Tie Grip

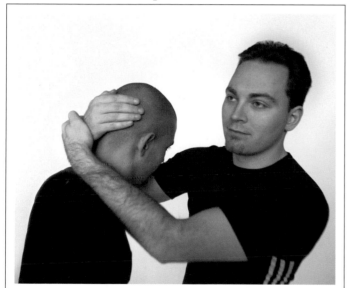

- There are several grips for the double neck tie grip, each with its own advantages.

- Placing one hand over the other is the easiest grip to achieve.

- Clasping palm to palm and squeezing the forearms together generate the most inward pressure.

- Placing a palm on the "bald spot" and hooking four fingers around your wrist controls the head well.

- Do not interlace your fingers. They can be injured as a result.

Pulling the Head Down

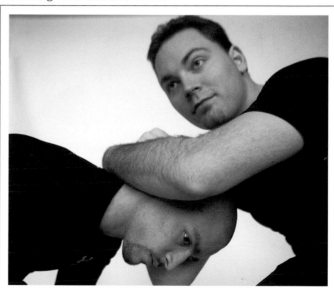

- When the double neck tie is established with both arms inside your attacker's arms, this strong position allows you to pull down on the head.

- Pulling his head down makes it much harder for your attacker to get away or to avoid strikes.

- The most common strike here is the knee, to the groin, thigh, or head (if it has been pulled low enough).

- Controlling the head and hitting it with many quick, powerful knee strikes are a potentially fight-ending tactic.

INTEGRATING THE FOUR HANDLES

The grips are most powerful in combination with each other and with other skills

With our four primary handles identified—wrist, bicep, underhook, and neck tie—we must look at their integration for use.

The handles of the clinch are meant to be used in conjunction with each other. Many of them can be used to counter each other. In fact, it is quite likely that at any point during the clinch phase, you may be controlling one handle with your left hand and a different one with your right; although you can establish double underhooks or double neck ties, it's more likely you'll have one of each simultaneously.

Regardless of the handles you're using at any given second, certain principles apply throughout. For starters you will

Neck and Bicep

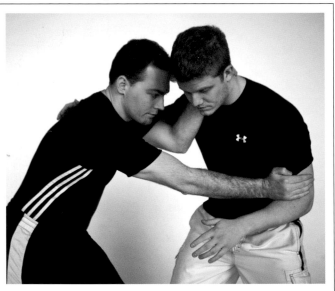

- One common combination of handles is the neck tie and bicep control.

- This position is easy to reach and is good for controlling the head while preventing punches.

- This position leaves one of your attacker's arms free, so you should continue driving forward to keep him off balance.

- Here you can throw strikes using both legs or quickly punch and then return to bicep control.

Underhook and Wrist

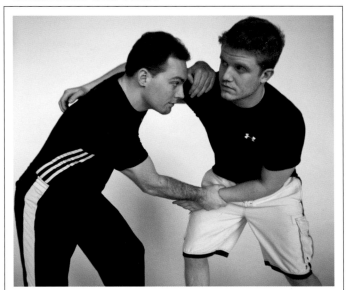

- Another common combination of controls is an underhook paired with wrist control.

- The underhook here prevents attempts at grabbing your legs, while the wrist control stops strikes on the far side.

- This can be used as a transition to establishing underhooks on both sides.

- This combination often suits shorter people wrestling with a taller opponent.

nearly always be driving forward, applying pressure to keep your assailant off balance.

Additionally, you'll want to seek the inside position with all the handles (except the wrist) because doing so gives you more direct access to the center of the body (and denies your attacker that control over you).

We can use many secondary clinch handles, but these four should be our primary foundation. Without any of these four, it would be almost impossible to establish solid control.

MAKE IT EASY

After we have established control in the clinch, we will—in most cases—move quickly into striking. Some of the most damaging tools are thrown at this close range, including elbowing the head, thumbing the eye, grabbing the groin, and kneeing the head, thigh, and groin. Our goal is typically to do enough damage to take the fight out of our attacker—or to take our attacker out of the fight.

Neck and Underhook

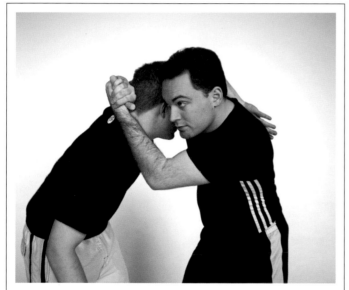

- The neck tie and underhook can be combined to control the shoulders and head.

- Sometimes in this position the hands are joined together, and the arms are squeezed—this position is known in wrestling as a "pinch headlock."

- The pinch headlock is a powerful control over the shoulders and, by extension, the arms. The inside arm feels stuck and can be hard to free.

- This is a great position for throwing knee strikes to the body.

Secondary Handles

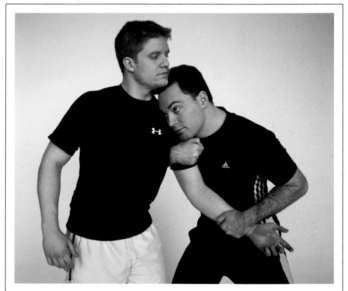

- There are many secondary methods of controlling the upper body in the clinch range.

- Many of these methods come from wrestling. The position pictured here is the "outside 2-on-1," which controls one arm with two while standing behind the opponent's arm.

- Secondary arm controls can be just as effective as the four primary handles, but they are less essential.

- The big four—wrist, bicep, underhook, and neck tie—are indispensable.

ENTERING CAUTIOUSLY
Make contact in a nonthreatening way in order to survey the scene

Sometimes you need to get closer to someone who appears agitated or confused, and you need a safe way to do it. The cautious entry is a safe, nonthreatening way to approach someone in order to intervene and take control of the situation.

In the cautious entry we place our hands, relaxed and palms forward, in the direct lines between our own face and the other person's biceps. This means that any attempt to grab or hit us will have to go around our hands, making the bicep control available to us in the process.

As we move forward to meet this person, we keep our arms in that position until we finally make contact with the biceps. In this way we keep ourselves protected the entire time.

One of the key features of this method is that it does not show any aggressive intent. With our hands up, palms forward, we send a message with our body language that we

Preparing to Enter

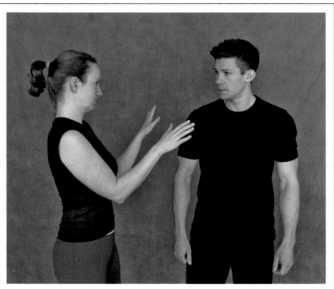

- The cautious entry is a nonaggressive, nonthreatening way to engage with someone who may or may not be a threat.

- The cautious entry is useful when we don't yet know if this person is hostile.

- This body language communicates to the person that you are not trying to escalate the situation.

- It's important to see that this method of engaging is also one that looks nonaggressive to other people who may be watching.

Hand Positioning

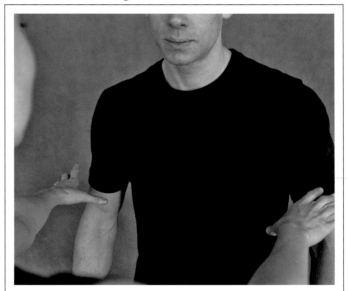

- The hand positioning for the cautious entry is specific and critical.

- The hands are placed in the direct lines between your chin and the other person's biceps.

- If the person suddenly becomes violent and attempts to hit or grab you, you will be able to defend strikes and establish bicep control.

- Keep your own elbows tucked in, as you would if you were already controlling the arms.

are trying to calm the other person and deescalate the situation. It's important that this message transmits appropriately both to the other person and to anyone watching, so we are not mistaken for the aggressor.

CONTROLLING DISTANCE

Approaching Contact

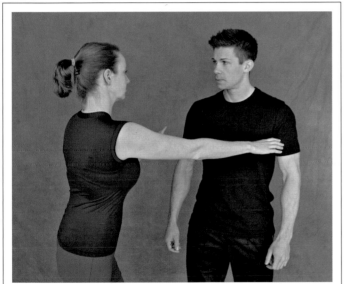

- As you make your approach with the cautious entry, monitor the other person's body language for signs of aggression.

- Keep your own body calm and relaxed and move forward confidently.

- Bring one side of your body forward as you near contact in case you will need to drive your weight into the bicep controls.

Contact and Interview

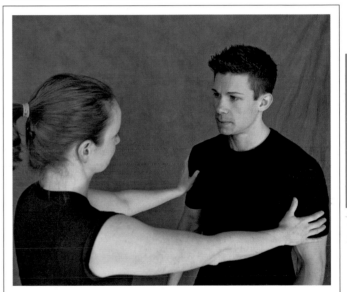

- Upon arriving at physical contact using the cautious entry, you can assess this person's mental state and see what should happen next.

- If the person is violent and enraged, you have the opportunity to continue controlling the arms and go onto to further measures.

- The cautious entry is not a step that commits you to a fight: If the person is confused or in need of assistance, you can use the contact made at the arms to help comfort and pacify him.

ENTERING AGGRESSIVELY
When strikes are already being thrown, you take a more direct approach to making contact

There are times when we need to get close to someone in order to end a situation now. One of the quickest methods of entering into the clinch range is the aggressive entry. This technique offers us reasonable protection against punches as we rush toward our attacker.

The aggressive entry is done at a sprint. You cover your head

with your arms, making sure that you can see between your arms, and run as fast as you can into your assailant. Because we cannot protect ourselves completely against strikes, we offer him the smallest window of time possible to hit us.

Cover yourself with your forearms and tuck your chin down. Close your mouth so that it won't slam shut upon impact.

Covering Up

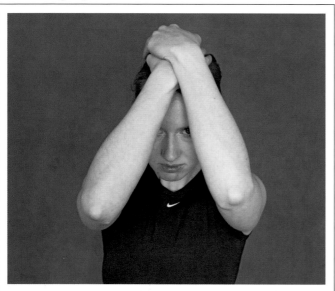

- Protect your head by placing both palms on the top of your head, overlapping.

- Squeeze your elbows downward and toward your body.

- Make sure that you can see down the center between your arms.

- Shrug your shoulders up and bring your chin down into your chest.

Running Forward

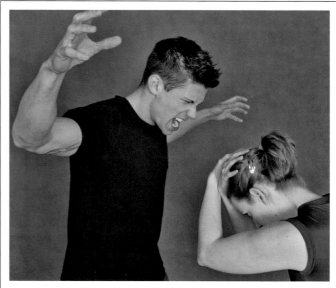

- With your head covered, enter as quickly as possible by running straight at your attacker.

- Aim your forearms (and forehead) at the center of the chest and run as fast as you can.

- The cover will diminish impact if your assailant tries to strike you as you run forward, but it cannot offer full protection.

- Don't waste time. Run at your attacker as quickly as possible to minimize the chance of being hit on your way in.

Your goal is to drive into your partner like a battering ram, using your head and arms. If you run quickly and hit solidly, you may even knock him off balance. Good. That will make it easier to establish control.

When you feel your arms and head make impact with his chest, quickly establish control in the clinch using the four major handles. Work quickly in order to maximize any advantage you may have gained when you rammed him.

ZOOM

One of the hardest things to do mentally is to decide to close the gap between you and someone violent. Remember that entering takes guts because it potentially places you in harm's way. Minimize the risk by moving as quickly as possible. Do not hesitate. Do not change your mind. Aim yourself directly at your opponent and then pull the trigger. Run. *Now.*

Entering inside a Punch

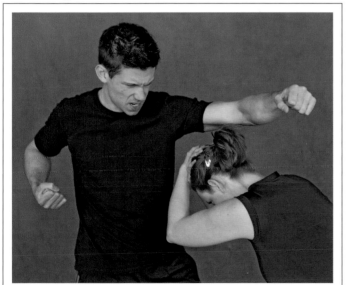

- Safety comes from being too far from the punches or inside the arc of haymaker-style punches. Don't waste any time when you're in between those distances.

- Time your run to minimize your vulnerability to punches, but don't wait long.

- You may not be able to avoid all of them, but the cover will offer some amount of protection as you sprint forward.

Contact

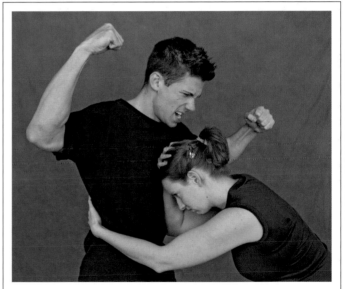

- Continue running forward until you feel your forearms make impact with your attacker's chest.

- Release the cover after you've made contact and immediately look to establish control using your four clinch handles.

- Tie up the arms and stop the attacker from throwing more punches.

- The forward pressure does not end when you make contact. Use the momentum to keep driving forward!

CONTROLLING DISTANCE

ENTERING FROM A STRIKE

Our safest opportunities to clinch often occur after a successful attack

The safest opportunity to grab someone is often right after we've hit him squarely. In particular, if we've hit a delicate area, we can capitalize on a split-second opportunity to take the advantage.

Hitting one of the primary targets (eye, throat, groin, or knee) is one of the more reliable ways to create a predictable,

instinctive reaction. Most people, when hit in one of these areas, bring their hands and attention to the area, even if only for a second. During that small window of time, we can rush forward and keep the momentum going in our favor.

Don't waste any time upon entering into range; start hitting right away. It's a good idea to throw strikes even in the

Eye Jab to Clinch 1

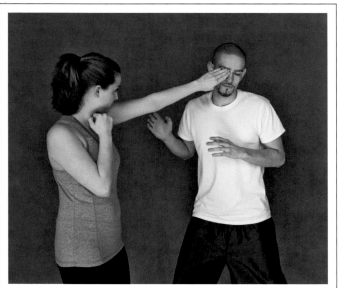

- A strike to the eye nearly always buys you a short window of time for action.

- In some cases it's clear that you need to make an entry to control this person and deliver some strikes, so you can use the eye jab to create time to enter.

- When you feel the eye jab make contact, and you see the expected reaction (hands to the eye), you have created a split second with a low risk of counterattack.

- Watch carefully for your window and be ready to act.

Eye Jab to Clinch 2

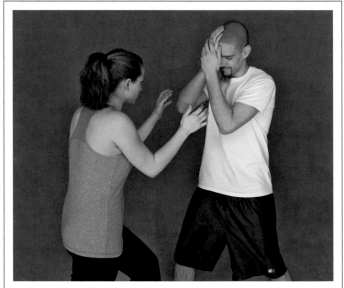

- When you see the hands go toward the face, you must act immediately.

- Make contact however you can. With the arms raised, the opportunity to drive forward and establish underhooks is increased.

- Depending on the position of the arms, you may be able to grab the neck tie.

- If you cannot establish control, you could throw the kick to the groin or another strong attack to try to increase your window of time.

second that you move forward into the clinch. Because our primary strategy is to overwhelm the opponent with a relentless flurry of strikes, we can exploit that moment of distraction to immediately use our strongest striking tools.

If more hitting is inappropriate to the situation, move to quickly and instantly overwhelm the opponent with your clinch controls. Drive into him without a second of hesitation. Plow him over and do not relinquish the advantage.

ZOOM

One of the trickiest skills to develop is the ability to see—in the chaos of fighting—a split-second window of time and to act upon it. This can take practice and experience, but above all it takes aggression. Any moment of opportunity given by our attacker should be our cue to release the floodgates and seize control of the situation.

Groin Kick to Clinch 1

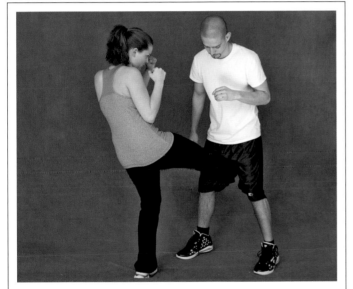

- The groin kick is another attack that can often create predictable reactions.

- If you need a second or two on your way to the clinch, this kick can provide the safety you need.

- On impact watch for the hips to push backward and the hands to come down. You're looking for these signs that your attack landed effectively and that you have a second or two to act.

- Be ready. Although these reactions are instinctive, they may not last long.

Groin Kick to Clinch 2

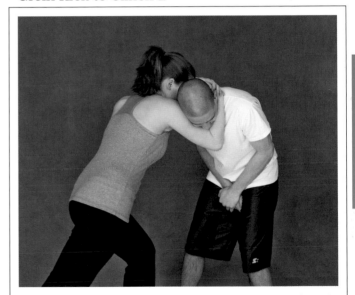

- When the hands move to the groin as a response to your attack, you have another opportunity to clinch strongly.

- His arms should be out of your way, and his head may be forward and down already.

- Make the grab quickly and begin throwing additional strikes, such as knees to the head.

- Don't give the attacker time to recover. Your goal is to overwhelm with the speed and fury of your counterattack.

GRABBED FROM THE FRONT

Take control by using your clinch handles when an attacker grabs you

When an attacker grabs you, he is attempting to control the situation by controlling you. Although grabs aren't very harmful by themselves, they are used to remove you from the scene or to hold you still for hitting or other reasons.

Although you are likely at a strength disadvantage against a grab (because few people attack someone stronger than themselves), you can still use the situation to your advantage. Because you understand the proper handles for effective control, you can turn this into an opportunity to take control of the attacker and the situation.

Depending upon how you've been grabbed, it may be less difficult or more difficult to find the room to move and

Bear Hug—Trapped Arms

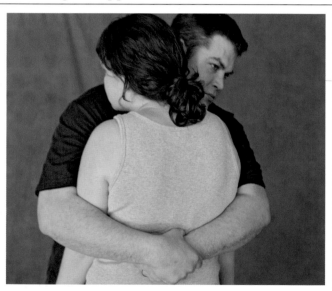

- One primitive method of fighting is to grab around the body with both arms and squeeze.

- The "bear hug" is a way by which some folks, often bigger and stronger people, try to establish control.

- Sometimes this is done in order to drag you away from your current location.

- When the bear hug is over your arms, they can be difficult to move.

Driving the Arms Up

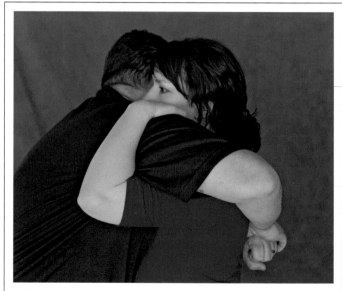

- If your arms are pinned underneath, drive your hips forward and push your arms around your opponent's body.

- Drive the arms up, either one at a time or simultaneously, and establish underhooks at the shoulders.

- By doing this, you take advantage of the opportunity given to you. This person has yielded the valuable "underneath" position of the arms; take it and establish control.

- As soon as you have more control, begin striking.

establish dominance. If he grabs you at arm's length, such as with a hair grab or a grab on the shoulder, you will have less difficulty establishing control. If the grab is tighter, such as a bear hug around the body, it may be difficult to move your arms into an advantageous position.

Sometimes it can be tricky if someone grabs your clothing or hair or is very strong. Anytime you need an extra advantage, strike at vulnerable areas while you're wrestling for control.

CONTROLLING DISTANCE

Bear Hug—Swim Under

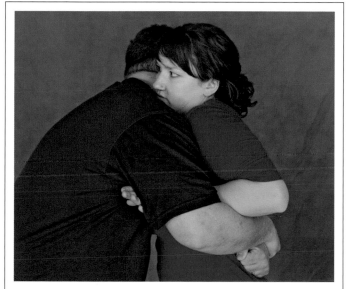

- Some bear hugs will go underneath your arms, leaving yours stuck on top.

- Here you've yielded the inside (underneath) position that gives you better control.

- In order to reestablish control, one option is to swim the arms back underneath.

- Turn your chest to the side, insert your hand through the front of his armpit, and drive your arm under.

- After you have one underhook, turn the other way and insert the opposite arm, too.

Bear Hug—Neck Tie

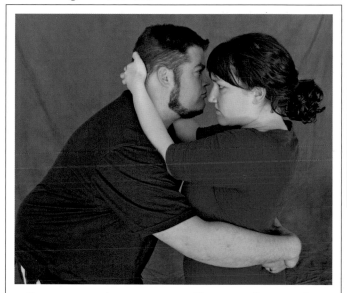

- If you cannot swim your arms back underneath, you have another option for taking control: Because your arms are on top, you can establish the neck tie.

- The hardest part is to create the space to get your elbows between your chest and his.

- Place your elbows on the front of his collarbones and wiggle them down between the two of you.

- Grab the back of the neck and drive your elbows forward to create separation and help break the bear hug.

GRABBED FROM BEHIND
Even these situations provide you the opportunity to establish control

Most attackers look for any advantage they can find. They will make an effort to surprise you, to catch you off guard, to give themselves control, and to make it harder for you to respond.

When you are grabbed from behind, the first priority is to reclaim your balance. This is especially true if you've been lifted off the ground. One of your priorities is to make sure you're not dragged to the ground. The next goal is to turn and get yourself facing your attacker. If you're standing still or being pushed forward, work to place one of your feet in front of you as a brace. This brace provides an opportunity to turn back into your attacker.

Even if you can turn only partway, try to wiggle one of your

Bear Hug—Behind 1

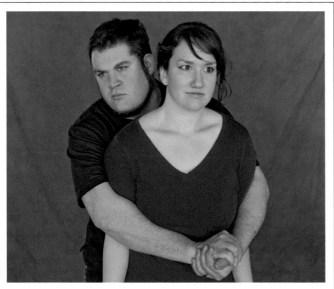

- Being grabbed from behind is a difficult situation because your eyes, arms, and legs are designed to work best in front of you.

- If your arms are above his, you can throw your elbows to the rear. With the arms pinned, this is much more difficult.

- One option is to immediately strike the groin with one or both hands. Doing this can buy you time and opportunity to improve your position.

Bear Hug—Behind 2

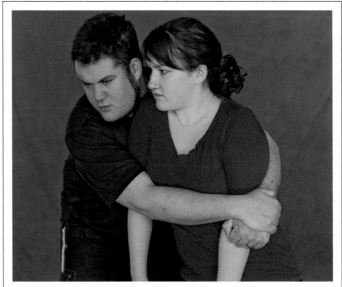

- When you feel that you have sufficient balance, take a step forward and plant your foot firmly into the ground.

- Pushing off that foot, turn abruptly to face your attacker. Although he may maintain his grip, you will be able to turn underneath his arms.

- It may take a couple of attempts to turn completely. That's okay. Turning to face him is a priority, so it's worth a few attempts.

arms through the narrow space between you and your assailant. Doing this allows you to fully turn to face him, negating the advantage of his having grabbed you from behind. Don't be delicate about it: push, pull, shove, and work that shoulder between the two of you so that you can turn around.

After you're facing your attacker, immediately establish control. If you're not hitting him already, begin right away.

CONTROLLING DISTANCE

Bear Hug—Behind 3

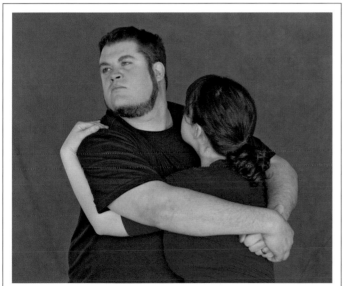

- After you've turned in to face your attacker, you now have the opportunity to establish control.

- Continue driving from the foot that helped you turn around and push yourself forward into your attacker.

- Drive both arms up underneath the armpits and establish your underhook control at the shoulders.

- Make sure you continue driving forward to make it harder for him to fight back.

Bear Hug Behind—Lifted

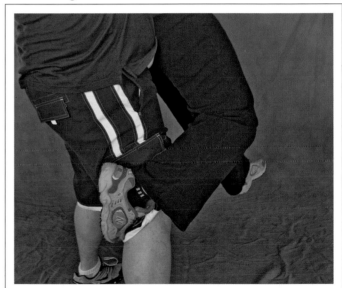

- When you are grabbed from behind, one risk is that your assailant will try to lift you from the ground.

- Use one of your legs to wrap around the outside of his. Hook the top of your foot securely in the back of the knee and pull your knee to your chest. This will

pull you back toward the ground, even against a big, strong attacker.

- Be sure to have your other foot ready to catch your balance as you return to the ground.

KEEPING YOUR DISTANCE
Maintain space when you'd prefer to avoid the clinch

In many situations it's better to avoid close quarters if you can. Sometimes you already have significant space between yourself and your attacker, and you should aim to keep it that way. Whether he tries to grab your upper body or lower body, there are some concepts you can use to keep him away if he tries to wrestle with you.

There are two important priorities when you're avoiding being grabbed: The first is to keep his shoulders away. If you let him close enough to grab with his arms, you're in for a struggle. Keep his shoulders at arm's length by pushing on the neck or side of the head. Try to steer him away from you rather than holding him back. If he tries to come in under your arms, you can push on both sides at once.

The second priority is to make it difficult for him to chase you. If he takes a running start, you don't want to stand still—he will have too much momentum for you to overcome.

Attempted Grab

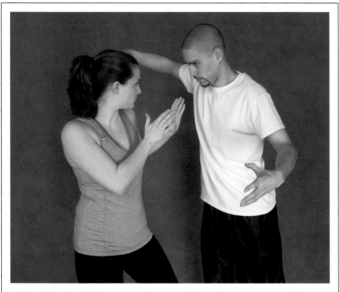

- Reading body language is important because the earlier you act, the better your options.

- When an attacker comes forwards to grab you, it's important that you don't stand still and allow it to happen.

- You also want to avoid backing up in a straight line. Although doing so feels natural, it allows your assailant to develop momentum as he walks or runs toward you.

Pushing and Circling

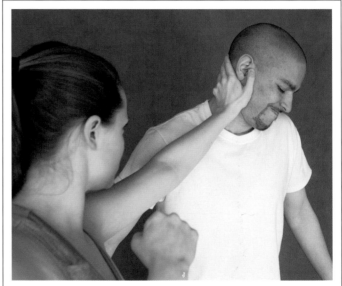

- Pick a direction and move in a circle to avoid your assailant. This makes it harder for him to chase you.

- Additionally, you can make it harder for him to grab you by pushing his head or neck away as you circle.

- If you're circling left, use your left hand to push. Likewise, push with your right when circling to the right. It keeps him away from the center of your body.

Avoid backing up for the same reason; it lets him pick up speed and momentum. Instead circle around him as you push against the head, neck, and shoulders. Try to steer him off course as you move your body in the opposite direction.

MAKE IT EASY

One common principle in the martial arts is to avoid fighting force on force when directly opposed. Even if you can win, it expends too much energy. When possible, avoid your opponent's force altogether. If a boulder rolls down a mountain at you, do you try to push it back, or do you move out of the way?

Punching and Circling

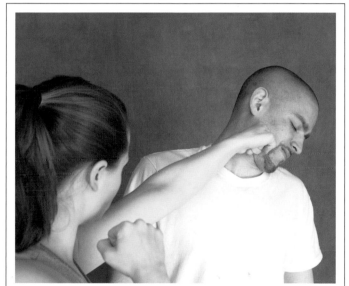

- While circling away from an attempted grab, you can also substitute a punch for the push.

- Try to aim your punch for the side of the jaw as you circle. Be careful not to hit the thick bones at the back of the head or above the ear with your fist—you're more likely to injure yourself.

- Throw your punch stiffly and firmly, so that it also pushes your assailant away.

Defending the Takedown

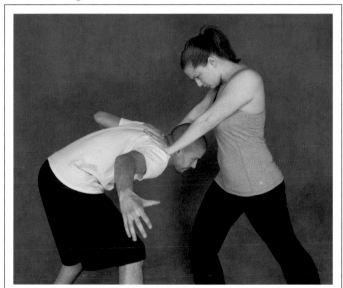

- If you cannot circle, you can stop the attacker from grabbing you by pushing both shoulders.

- Keep his chest and shoulders away from you by pushing on them with both hands. In a tight space, you can push with your forearms.

- This method of defense also works if he attempts to grab you around the waist or legs.

- With your arms committed, you can still throw kicks and knees to help take the advantage.

HAIR PULLING
A grip on the hair can be a useful handle for controlling your attacker

Gripping the hair can be a great tool both for causing pain and for controlling your attacker in close quarters. We can use a grip on the hair to manipulate the head, whether we're creating opportunities to strike or to move.

Although hair pulling isn't something we can use to finish a fight all by itself, it works well in conjunction with our other close-range tactics. We can grab the hair as a handle for control, and it can be a very secure grip, depending on how long the attacker's hair is. Dig your fingers in until you reach the scalp and then close them around a big fistful of hair. You can often find the best grip on the top of the head or at the back corners of the head. If your attacker has longer hair, it will be

Pulling the Hair

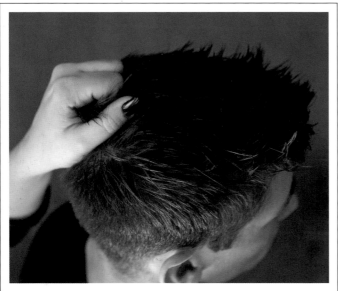

- Pulling the hair can be a good tool for controlling the head and creating space.

- The most secure hair pull grabs the hair on the top of the head and pulls the head straight backward.

- Even when hair is short, the hair on the top is often the easiest to grab. Get a good, secure grip on it.

- In addition to providing control, a hair grab is also painful.

Turning the Head

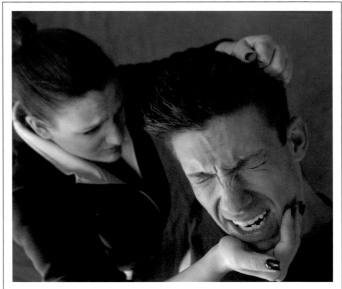

- You can also turn the head by controlling it with the hair.

- One of the strongest ways to do this is to grab the hair on the back corner of the head and to place your palm on the near side of the chin.

- Push on the chin as you pull the hair to turn the head strongly and securely.

- Turning the head in this way is difficult to fight against and can be used to separate yourself from your attacker.

easier to take hold, but you should still look to grab it along the scalp instead of farther down.

We can also pair hair pulling with striking and other close-range options. With a secure grip on the hair, you can punch or elbow the face, pulling the head into your strikes as you throw them. You can also use the hair grab to hold the head still for a moment while you thumb the eye or bite. Or you can use your grip on the hair to pull the head down into a knee strike.

Additionally, we can integrate the hair pull with our clinch handles. In particular the neck tie can be performed with a full grip on the hair, making it difficult to escape. In some cases we can also use the hair pull when we need to pull our attacker away from us but cannot get our arms into position for our primary handles.

Neck Tie Using Hair

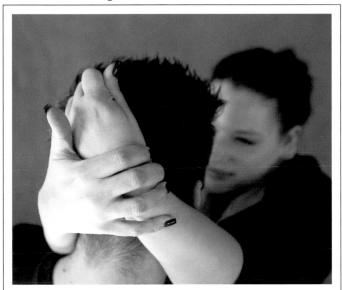

- You can create a secure variation of the neck tie control by using the hair.

- Grip the hair at the back of the head firmly and drive your forearm under the jawbone.

- Grab your own wrist with your free hand and squeeze your elbows together.

- This grip affords more control over the head than the standard neck tie and creates pain and distraction.

Striking with Hair Pull

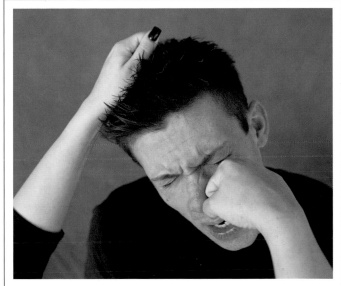

- Controlling the head by holding the hair is a great way to create opportunities for strikes.

- Hold the head and move it into any punches, elbows, knees, or kicks that you throw. The strikes will be much harder for your assailant to avoid.

- If your attacker has long hair, you can also grab a ponytail or a fistful of hair for the same purposes.

ELBOWS
The elbows are solid striking tools when you are too close to punch

The elbows are a great striking tool in close quarters because they are a solid surface that resists injury and can be thrown with tremendous power.

We can make two types of impacts with the elbow: We can aim the bony tip of the elbow, or we can hit with the broad side of the forearm. Each is good for different cases.

With the tip of the elbow, we can strike with great power at narrow areas. The tip of the elbow can break the skin,

especially when it connects with the head or face, leaving the attacker cut and bloodied.

On the other hand, we can also throw strikes with the fleshy side of the forearm, which has a broader area and creates a more concussive impact. This strike can be thrown effectively even when we target hard, bony areas such as the back of the head and neck or the bridge of the nose.

Elbows are delivered like punches: The body rotates and

Horizontal Elbow Strikes

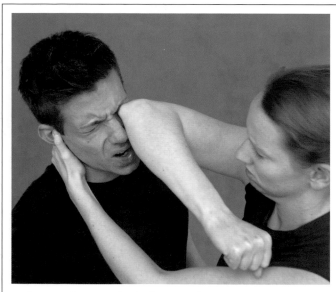

- The most basic method of throwing the elbow is from side to side, hitting a target in front of you.

- You can deliver a "football-style" elbow strike by pushing forward with the forearm, or you can strike with the tip of the elbow for a focused impact.

- Elbows can be powerful because of their small striking surface. They often cause cuts if they strike the face or head.

Rearward Elbows

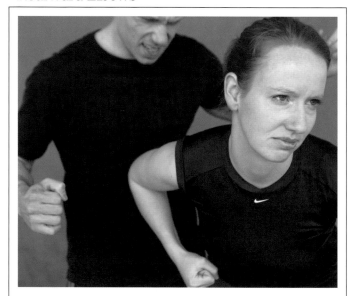

- The elbow is a versatile tool because it can be thrown behind you as easily as it can be thrown forward.

- When grabbed from behind, you can throw an elbow to the solar plexus, striking anywhere available on the abdomen.

- With your arms on top, you could also throw the rearward elbow to the head.

- Rearward elbows are driven by the muscles of the back, which are large and powerful.

pushes off of both legs, driving your hips (and therefore weight) into the strike. They are immensely powerful and can be thrown in great numbers very quickly.

Elbows can also be thrown at any angle you can imagine: up, down, backward, and diagonally. They are an excellent tool in close quarters.

Descending Elbows

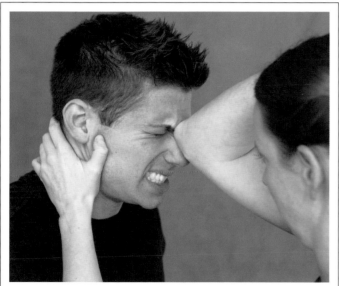

- In close quarters or ground-fighting situations, you may have an opportunity to throw a strike downward using the bony tip of the elbow.

- These strikes are best targeted to the face, neck, or other delicate areas.

- It can be hard to be precise when throwing this kind of strike. Aim for big targets.

Ascending Elbows

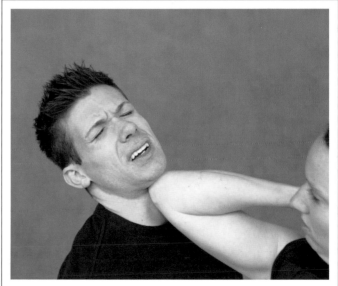

- In some situations you can also throw the elbow strike upward.

- This strike is often thrown to the chin, knocking the head backward and slamming the jaw shut.

- In situations when someone is standing over you, this kind of strike can also target the groin.

CLOSE-RANGE STRIKING

99

HEADBUTTING

When the arms are unavailable, the head is another solid striking tool

Another tool for extremely close-range combat is the head-butt. Often it happens unintentionally in the clinch. It's important that when you use the head for striking, you injure your attacker but not yourself.

The strongest surfaces of the head are the back, the top, and the border where the forehead meets the crown of the head. These should be your primary striking surfaces when you headbutt.

The headbutt can be thrown in many directions. You can throw it backward at someone who has grabbed you from behind or forward if you are face to face. If you are shorter than your attacker, you can drive your head upward below

Headbutt Forward

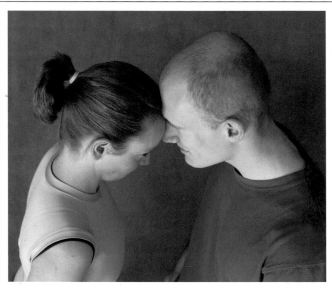

- The simplest headbutt travels forward, using the line between the forehead and the top of the head.

- This strike is commonly thrown to the nose, especially when both people are similar in height.

- Be sure to close your own teeth when you headbutt. If your jaw slams closed from the impact, you could give yourself a concussion.

Headbutt Sideways

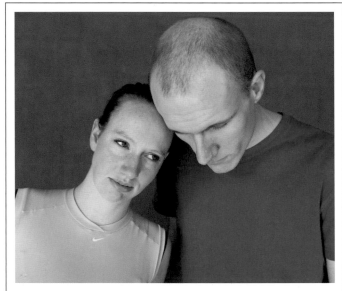

- Headbutts can also be thrown at an angle, using the front corner of the head.

- Be sure to avoid striking your temple next to the eye. On the other hand, it's a great target on your attacker. You can also aim for the nose.

- If you find yourself stuck very close to your attacker, you can deliver a short, sharp strike in this way to the side or middle of the face.

the chin or directly into his nose. If the two of you are similar in height, you can strike the nose or temple (the side of the forehead) with the crown of your head.

Headbutts can be thrown as short, surprising strikes, or you can use your legs to drive forward (or upward) into a much stronger, more deliberate headbutt. Each of these methods has its advantages at close range.

• • • • • • • • • • • • RED ● LIGHT • • • • • • • • • • • • • •
When headbutting, it's important to clench your teeth. If your jaw is open on impact, it can cause your teeth to slam shut, which can give you a concussion (as well as injure your jaw). To prevent this danger, keep your teeth firmly together anytime you strike with your head.

Full-crown Headbutt

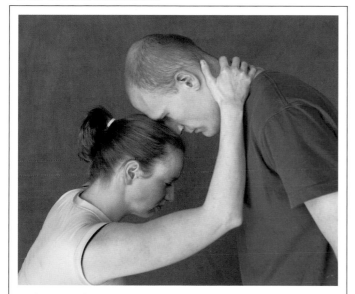

- The most devastating headbutt is thrown with the entire top of the head. Close your teeth and drive your head forward into the target.

- This headbutt, much like the others, is best delivered directly to the face. Targeting the nose or other weak structures is ideal.

- Be sure to hit your target straight on to avoid injuring your neck.

- Drive with both legs as you throw this headbutt. If you have control of your opponent's neck, pull him into the strike.

Headbutting Backward

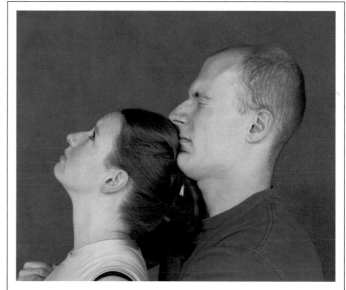

- The headbutt can also be thrown to a target behind you.

- Close your teeth and swing the head back, striking with the back part of the skull.

- This can be a surprising attack to someone who is holding you from behind, even on the ground.

- Though you cannot see where your head is going, your goal is to strike the nose.

CLOSE-RANGE STRIKING

101

BITING
Create space, pain, and panic using a visceral tool

When you find yourself trapped close to your attacker, one of the best tools in your arsenal is the bite.

Biting causes immense pain, especially when it's done to sensitive areas. It can target almost any part of the body, but some particularly good ones are hands and fingers, the upper arm, the side of the neck, the face, the nipple, the inside thigh, and the groin.

Although all of these areas are sensitive, some of them, such as the side of the face and neck, will cause immense panic. Most people don't expect such a vicious response—having someone sink her teeth into you can be scary!

When we bite, our goal is not to draw blood. Rather we perform many quick, aggressive, sharp bites—like a piranha—to cause as much pain as possible.

One reason why the bite works as a self-defense tool is because it causes the attacker to panic. We want him to

Bite the Arm

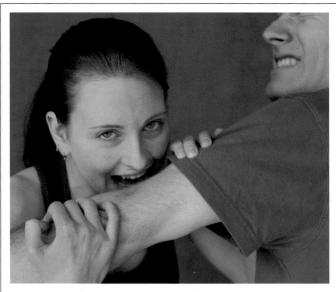

- When wrestling in the clinch range, one of the easiest targets to bite is the upper arm.

- When your attacker grabs you or pushes you, take hold of the arm and bring it to your mouth.

- Bite sharply, like a strong pinch. Bites should be quick and repeated.

- Your goal is to make him pull the arm away, not to draw blood.

Bite the Hand

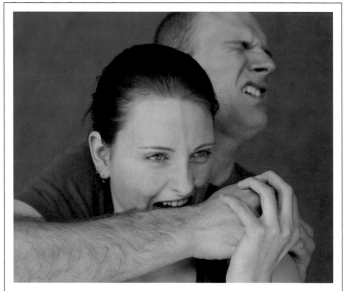

- When you are grabbed from behind, your assailant's hands or forearms may be available to bite.

- If an arm is near your neck or face, bring it to your teeth with your hands.

- Bite sensitive areas such as the fingers and hands. Doing this will make him more likely to let go in order to protect himself.

- If he covers your mouth with his hand, bite it!

realize that this assault was the worst decision he has ever made, and we want him to regret it in an instant. Few things will cause him to panic and change his mind as quickly as feeling several fast, vicious bites on the side of his face.

Bite the Body

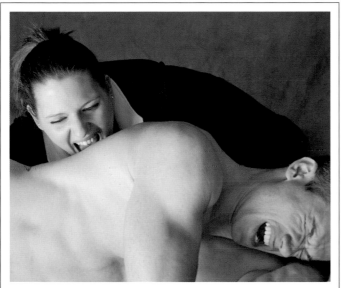

- The side of the body is another sensitive area.

- Bite along the ribs or the muscles of the back that form back of the armpit. To create intense pain, bite the nipple.

- In some ground-fighting situations, you may be within range to bite the inside thigh or even the groin. This can be an extremely effective method of escaping when pinned.

Bite the Face

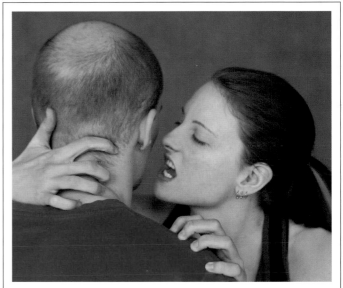

- When trapped up close, bite the side of the face or neck.

- As before, your goal is not to draw blood but rather to create intense pain. The side of the face and neck are extremely sensitive areas.

- You also intend to create panic, given the viciousness of your counterattack.

- Few people will choose to continue an assault in the face of an aggressive "victim" who will not stop biting their neck and face.

THUMB IN THE EYE

This is a good attack on a sensitive target in close quarters

In the clinch range one of the most easily accessible attacks is a thumb to the eye. Because you swim your hand behind the neck to establish the neck tie control, the eyes are an easy stop along the way. You can slide your hand into position to attack the eye very quickly and with little warning. Pulling on the back of the head or neck with your free hand can support the thumb attack and make it much harder to defend against or to move the head away.

Likewise, if you pull the head down while controlling the clinch or defending a takedown, you may get your fingers into the eye. Doing this can add some extra pain and disorientation while you take control of your attacker.

If you're holding a weapon or another object—even something simple like a pen, keys, or the mail—you can use your thumb to press it against the eye in the same manner.

Whether intentional or not, if you have foreign substances

Thumb in the Eye

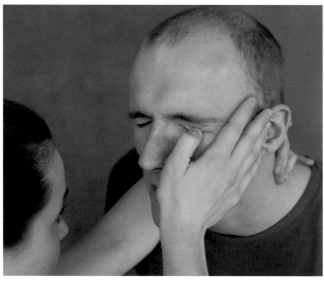

- When wrestling in the clinch range or on the ground, one of the easiest ways to attack the eye is to use your thumb.

- Press hard against the eye using the pad, tip, or nail of the thumb.

- You can also pull the eyelid closed and then press, all in one action.

- Controlling the back of the head or neck can make it easier to apply the thumb to the eye.

Thumbing to Escape

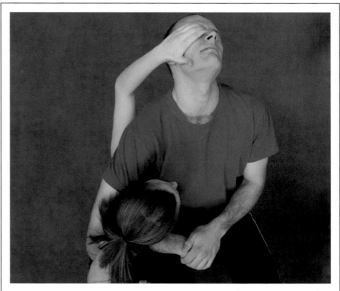

- In some situations you can use a thumb or finger to the eye to begin the process of escaping.

- A finger in the eye drives the head backward in addition to causing intense pain and distraction.

- When your attacker's arms are busy, this can be a great opportunity to direct your attack to the eye.

- Move quickly and attack strongly because your window of time may be brief.

(dirt, liquids, and so forth) on your thumb, you can rub them into the eye when you attack it. This transfer can cause a more intense or lasting pain and irritation.

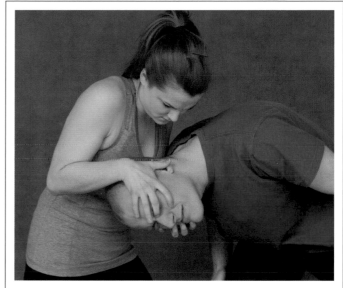

Biting and Gouging . . . Really?

- Many people consider these tactics a little gruesome and extreme.

- Remember to apply the following rule: "If I would do it in order to protect my mother, then it is a technique I should practice."

- By this standard you may be willing to bite someone or thumb the eye if necessary.

- However, you may not be willing to apply these tactics, and that's perfectly okay. Use the rule above to decide what you would and wouldn't do.

Fingers in the Eyes

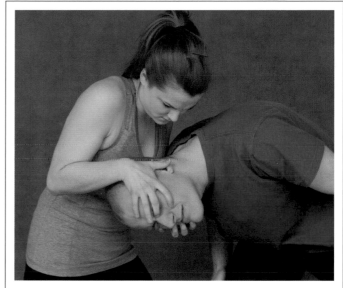

- Sometimes while controlling the head, there are incidental (if not accidental) opportunities to attack the eyes.

- Take advantage of the smallest opportunity to add pain and distraction.

- Splashing a drink into the eyes can be another irritant—especially if it's hot or contains alcohol.

- Even when the contact is only incidental, disturbing the eyes can buy you time to get away or to launch more significant attacks.

CLOSE-RANGE STRIKING

GROIN SLAP/GRAB
Close range presents many opportunities to attack the groin

When in the clinch range, you can attack the groin in a number of ways because it's within arm's length.

There are many opportunities to hit, slap, and grab the groin in the clinch. When you're wrestling for control, you can use your inside position at the bicep or the underhook to clear a path to hit the groin. At this close range, it's difficult for the attacker to see this strike coming or to defend it.

A successful groin shot can stun your attacker, making it easier for you to control him in the clinch. It can also buy you the time you need to fire several knees, elbows, or other finishing shots in order to neutralize the attack or make your exit.

Even if your groin attack doesn't land as intended, it can still get a flinch response. Most men will instinctively try to defend their groin, even if the hit isn't going to land. And if it does land, nearly every man will bring his hands there right away.

Slap the Groin

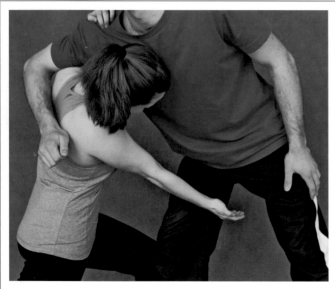

- The easiest attack to the groin in close quarters is a simple slap with the hand.

- When wrestling for control at the bicep or shoulder, the slap to the groin is readily available. As you swim your arms to the inside position, move quickly to the strike to the groin.

- Cup your hand as you strike, making impact with the palm and fingers. Hold the fingers together so that none of them is injured.

- Even if the slap misses, most men will flinch at any strike intended for the groin.

Grab the Groin

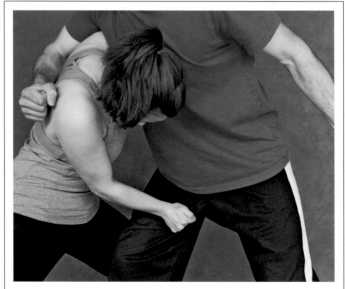

- When striking the groin, any slap can easily become a grab.

- The grab can also be used with a twisting or pulling action.

- A solid grip can cause tremendous pain. The testicles are an extremely sensitive target, and the pain response to grabbing or pulling is instantaneous and severe.

- Although primarily a tactic against men, slapping and grabbing the groin can also be an effective strike against a female attacker.

MAKE IT EASY

Depending on the situation, you can strike the groin in a number of ways: an open-handed slap, a grab, a punch, or a hammering strike with the top or bottom of the fist. Each of these has advantages, but the shortest answer is that it doesn't matter *how* you hit the groin; just hit it!

Striking with Your Fist

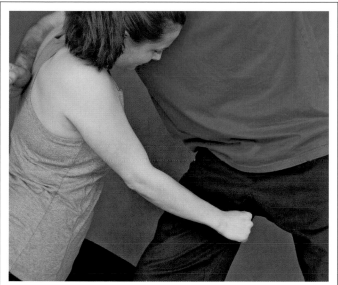

Attacked from Behind

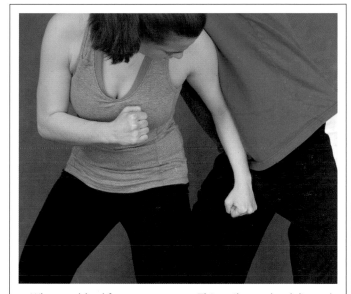

- Another method of attacking the groin is with the front of your fist.

- You can deliver a strike with the thumb side of the fist. Swing the entire hand forward, aiming with the knuckle at the base of the index finger.

- Be sure to tuck your thumb next to your fingers (but not inside your fist) so that you do not jam or dislocate it.

- When grabbed from behind, you can still slap or grab the groin.

- Swing your fist downward in a motion much like a hammer. As it reaches the bottom of its arc, make contact with the bottom side of the fist.

- This strike can be delivered with the fist or as an open-handed slap. In both cases it can be followed by a grab.

- Several quick, strong strikes such as this can be very effective.

CLOSE-RANGE STRIKING

PULLED BY THE ARM

Here's one example of dealing with an attempted grab

In this example sequence, we see an attacker begin with an abduction-style threat. He grabs our "victim," Meagin, by the arm and attempts to drag her away.

In comparison with chokes or hits, this pulling attack is a low-level threat, provided that Meagin can stop him from taking her from the scene.

In this case she responds by initially resisting and then uses the force of his pull to help her throw a hard right cross.

Because his hands are both committed, she can take the time to throw a solid, well-aimed punch, knowing he won't have a chance to block it. This punch begins the process of turning the tide in her favor.

Without hesitating she follows the right cross with a knee to the groin. She chooses the knee here because he may still have a hold of her arm—although he may also bring his hands up to his face. She's not waiting long enough to watch

Dragged by the Arm

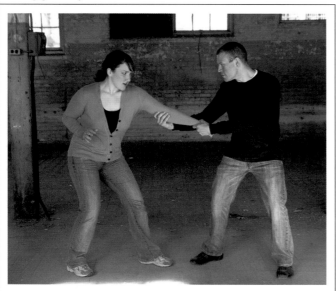

- In this example our attacker drags Meagin by the arm.

- Although the grab itself is a low-priority threat compared with strikes and chokes, the danger is the possibility of being removed from the scene.

- Situations become much more serious if you leave the initial scene. Statistically the odds of survival diminish radically.

- Here Meagin acts quickly before the situation becomes worse and more variables are outside her control.

Initial Response—Cross

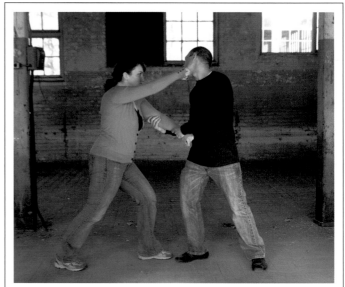

- Because her attacker's arms are committed to the grab, Meagin responds with a powerful attack with her free hand: a right cross to the face.

- It's crucial that she sets her feet in order to throw this punch with power. This is especially true when she's being pulled off balance.

- Meagin makes a good choice here, hitting with a strong attack during a moment when her assailant's face is unguarded.

what he does. It's a hard cross and then a step right into the knee for a quick 1-2.

After a few quick knees, his head comes down, so she grabs on to throw a knee to the head. When she sees him fall, she'll waste no time escaping to safety.

Knee to the Groin

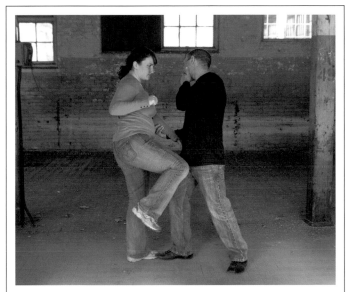

- After landing the right cross successfully, Meagin has a brief opportunity to initiate more substantial attacks.

- Regardless of whether her wrist arm is free yet, Meagin can throw the knee.

- She steps forward following the right cross and drives a knee to the groin. And if she can, she lands several of these in a row.

- These knees will buy her more time and maybe even end the confrontation.

Knee to the Head

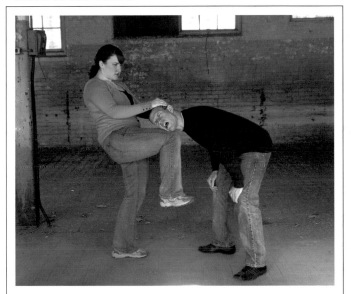

- Having freed her wrist, Meagin grabs a hold of her attacker's head.

- Because she landed the knees to the groin, her attacker's head is lower and within reach.

- Several strong knee strikes to the head take the fight out of her assailant. If they knock him to the ground, she'll take the opportunity to disengage and run.

SKILLS IN CONTEXT 1

CHOKE FROM THE FRONT
Defend a primal assault from an untrained attacker

Chokes are a higher priority of attack than grabs because they place you in danger right away. Here our "victim," Lena, must immediately dip her chin to protect her airway and deal with the grip on her neck right away.

Dealing with the pressure on the neck is an essential priority. She needs to protect the airway from the pressure of the thumbs squeezing against the front of the neck, which could cause her to pass out. If the pressure is also occluding the arteries on the sides of the neck, it is even more likely that she will not stay conscious long.

After her chin is down, Lena grabs a hold of her attacker's wrists. She uses a strong plucking motion, aided by the large muscle groups of her back to create space around her neck. At the same time she fires a knee to the groin, knowing that if her attacker is very strong, she will need the knee to help distract him and loosen his grip as she removes it.

Choke from the Front

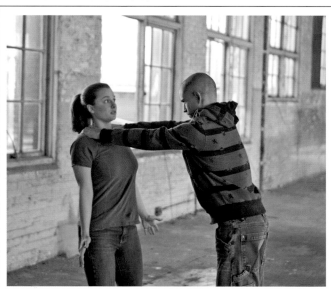

- Lena is attacked with a choke from the front. Chokes of this type are a primal, untrained attack.

- The danger here is the strength of the fingers squeezing the windpipe.

- It's a crude attack, but the danger is real.

- When the neck is attacked, the natural reflex is to bring your hands to your neck. You should use this reflex in your defense.

Releasing the Hands

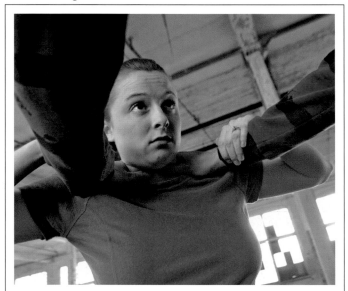

- Lena grabs over the top of the attacker's hands, hooking her fingers where the thumb meets the wrist.

- With a firm grip established, she drives her elbows down and back, using the strong muscles of her back. This pries the attacker's hands apart and away from her neck, releasing the pressure.

- It's important to use the strong muscles of the back rather than trying to lift with the arms.

- Be sure to grab right at the wrist—it's weaker than the upper arm.

She throws several knees, and when his hands go to his groin, she takes a grip on the neck and begins to throw elbows. She will continue throwing strong knee and elbow strikes in order to overwhelm him until she can make her exit.

Knee to the Groin

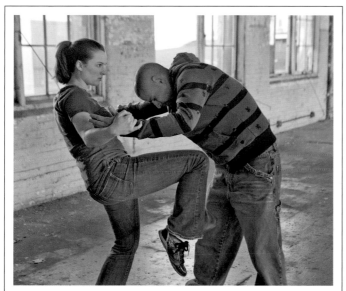

- As Lena clears the hands, she takes advantage of the fact that her attacker's hands are committed and throws a knee to the groin.

- The impact of the knee will help diminish the strength of the choke, helping facilitate the release.

- By launching the knee at the same time as her defense, Lena makes the most of her opportunity in case it's the only one she has.

- Also it should buy her time to launch into a complete counterassault.

Elbow to the Head

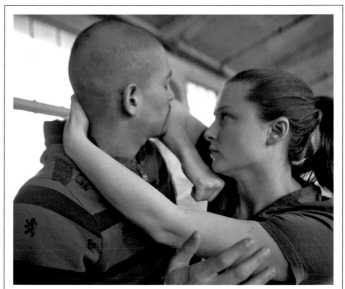

- Now that she has made an opportunity, Lena launches into a series of elbow strikes to the head.

- It's important that she doesn't hesitate during this critical second.

- Instead she should proceed right into a vicious

and powerful attack that will turn the tide before her assailant builds any momentum.

- She will continue her counterattack until she sees that the danger has passed or has an opportunity to disengage safely.

CHOKE FROM THE REAR 1
How to escape a surprise attack from behind

In this example Lena is grabbed in a surprise attack from the rear. Although chokes that rely on finger strength are crude and inefficient, her immediate reaction must still be to tuck her chin and protect her airway.

The next step is to dislodge the hands from her neck in order to turn and take control of her attacker face to face. She takes a step forward in order to establish her balance and raises her forearm so that her elbow is higher than his arms.

In an abrupt movement powered by the leg in front of her, she turns sharply to face him. As she does so, her raised arm will drive across and into his forearms, clearing them to the side and releasing his hands from her neck.

At the same time she sends her fist crashing down onto his nose. It's a surprising move because only fractions of a second earlier, she was facing away from him, and he was successfully choking her. If he was able to hold onto her neck

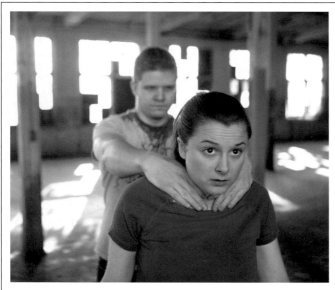

Choke from the Rear

- A choke from behind can be a scary threat because it can be difficult to reach the attacker.

- Chokes such as this one using the fingers are a primitive and inefficient method of attack but should still be dealt with seriously.

- Attacks from behind are usually used when someone is ambushed. In a situation such as this, it's unlikely you were aware of your assailant until the attack.

- Although this puts you at an automatic disadvantage, there are still effective techniques for this situation.

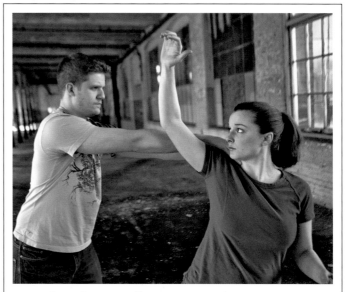

Preparing to Release

- In order to free yourself from the choke, you must first establish your balance and prepare your body to generate the right power.

- Step forward with one foot. If you are being pushed forward, this is essential in catching your balance.

- Even if you are stationary, you will want to stagger your stance in this way to prepare to turn.

- Whichever foot stepped forward, raise the opposite arm. It's important that your elbow reaches above the arms holding your neck.

even a little, the pain in his nose will distract him from it.

Seizing the brief moment of surprise, Lena steps forward and fires a series of knee strikes to the groin. As he collapses, she will push him away and make a safe escape.

Releasing the Choke

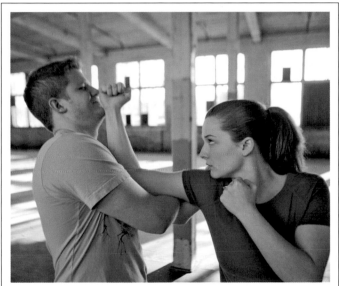

- Push off your forward foot and turn to face your attacker. Use the back of your tricep and your armpit to clear the hands.

- Turn sharply with a quick motion to break the grip. Although you may not disengage the hands completely, you should be able to release the pressure on your neck.

- As you turn, bring your elbow or fist down into your assailant's face. This will help to distract him as you release the choke, making it easier to break free.

Finishing with a Knee

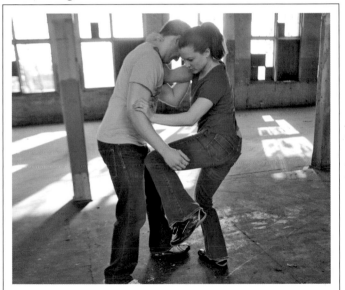

- Having struck a quick, distracting blow, you should immediately move into more severe measures.

- With the hands traveling to the face, the groin is left exposed. Here Lena follows up with a knee to the groin.

- Do not hesitate. Create the fraction of a second you need to turn the tide and then act quickly and decisively.

- It doesn't matter what targets you choose, but hit them swiftly and repeatedly.

SKILLS IN CONTEXT 1

CHOKE FROM THE REAR 2
Defend a stronger type of choking situation

Chokes performed with the forearm are a much more dangerous threat than those performed with the hands. Here we contend with greater strength and the sturdier structure of the arm (as opposed to the fingers). The risk in this kind of attack is much higher and needs immediate attention.

As the "victim," Morgan, feels the choke around her neck, she brings her chin down and grabs into the wrist with both hands. Rather than pulling on the upper arm or the elbow,

she hangs her weight on the wrist, where it will take the most strength to fight against her. To bring some pain and distraction to her aid, she stomps her heel onto the instep of her attacker's foot.

Feeling a little bit more room to move, she brings his arm in front of her face and bites the hand and forearm. She makes several sharp, quick bites along here until she feels him try to pull his arm away from her.

Choke with the Arm

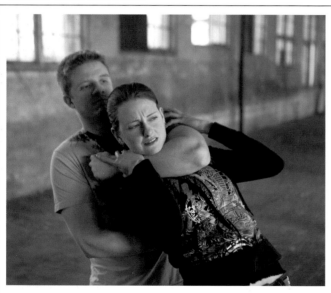

- A choke with the arm is a much more significant threat than chokes done with the hands and fingers.

- The arm is a strong structure that is capable of creating much more pressure on the neck.

- Against the front of the

neck, we worry about injury to the trachea.

- With pressure on the sides of the neck, blood flow to the brain is diminished, and unconsciousness comes quickly.

- This is a severe threat. You must act.

Creating an Opening

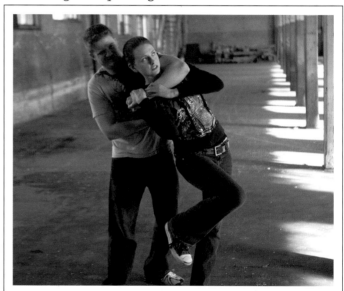

- Morgan feels the arm around her neck and instantly goes into action.

- She begins by grabbing the wrist to pry it away from her neck. The wrist will be the area where she can mount the most strength against the power of the arm.

- At the same time she stomps the foot to cause pain and distraction, taking her assailant's mind off of her attempt to peel off the arm.

When that happens, she feels the opportunity to improve to a better position to control him. She drives her shoulder back, into his chest and turns to face him. Here she blocks his far bicep in case he tries to grab or hit her, and she slides her other arm into an underhook position. The instant she establishes control, she will begin hitting.

Cause Him to Disengage

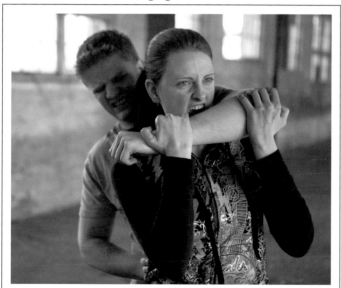

- Having created a little bit of space, Morgan takes a secure grip on the arm and brings it closer to her mouth.

- She bites anything she can: the fingers, the hand, the forearm. Morgan uses quick, sharp bites to cause tremendous pain on these sensitive areas.

- The goal is to make her attacker try to free his arm. If he's pulling the arm away from her, she's no longer in danger of being choked.

Establish Control

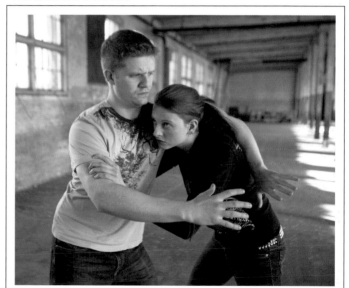

- Having taken the momentary advantage, Morgan turns to face her attacker and immediately drives forward.

- She establishes control quickly and ties up the arms, placing herself in a strong position so that not only has she removed the threat of another choke, but also she is now in a position to launch her own offensive.

- By creating a moment of pain and panic for her attacker, she has turned the tables and begun to control the scene.

SKILLS IN CONTEXT 1

LIFTED FROM BEHIND
Techniques for an attacker who carries you off of the ground

Being lifted from the ground is a vulnerable situation. We want to avoid being taken from the scene or being thrown to the ground.

Here the "victim," Lena, immediately hooks her leg behind her attacker's knee in order to keep him from lifting her any higher. With the foot hooked, she pulls her knee to her chest in order to bring herself back down to the ground safely, landing on her free foot.

As they land and their collective weight comes forward, she pushes both legs straight into the ground and fires a head-butt back into her attacker's face. Because she can't see him in this position, she chooses any easy target to hit without looking. Even if she doesn't hit his nose, she's bound to collide with some part of his head and cause him injury.

With his attention on his face, Lena brings one arm down and grabs the groin. While she pulls and twists to cause

Hook the Leg

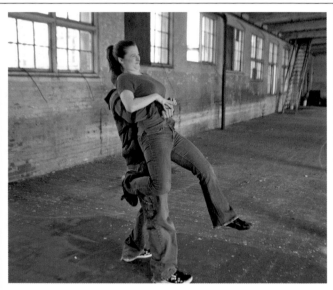

- Being lifted from the ground can be a dangerous proposition. This attack can be used to defend in an abduction situation or to bring you to a space in your environment where it's harder for you to fight back.

- Here Lena immediately hooks her leg backward around her assailant's to pull herself back down to the ground.

- She is careful to have her other leg ready to catch her balance as she approaches the ground.

Backward Headbutt

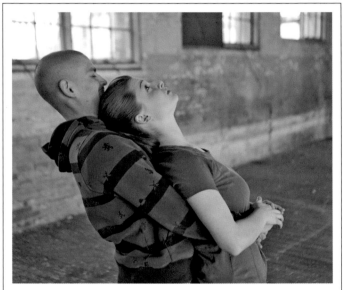

- Upon landing Lena wastes no time and immediately fires her head backward at her attacker.

- In order to throw this head-butt with power, she bends her legs and lowers her stance as soon as she's back on the ground.

- Having compressed her knees like springs, she drives up with both legs and sends her head crashing into his nose.

- She is careful to keep her own jaw closed as her head makes impact.

additional pain, she also turns her body to see him better. In this way she can judge the effectiveness her counterattacks are having, and she decides whether she can disengage or whether she will need to take firmer control.

As he reacts to the pain of the groin shot, and his grip around her loosens, Lena takes a step forward and fires a strong stomp to the front of his knee. From this position she can start running before he even hits the ground.

Grab the Groin

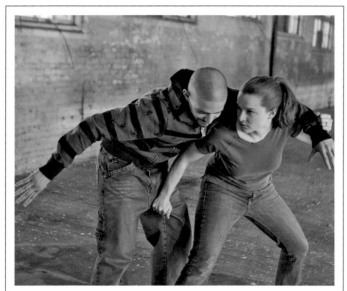

- Having created a brief distraction with the pain of the headbutt, Lena reaches down and grabs him by the groin.

- Between the headbutt and the groin attack, his grip is weakened. She steps forward to begin turning to face him, although she still has a hold of the groin.

- Lena puts these attacks together at a rapid pace, with no wasted time between them.

Attack the Knee

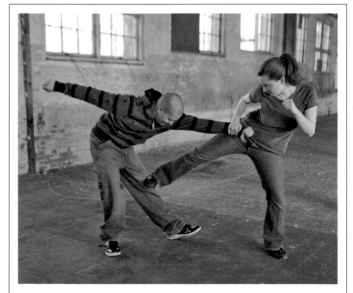

- With room to turn and begin to separate herself from her attacker, Lena releases her grip on the groin and fires a stomp to the kneecap, hoping to cause pain and injury to the knee.

- Lena hopes to cause an injury to the knee with her stomp or, at the least, to knock her assailant down.

- Even if the effect is only temporary, the stomp can buy her the time and opportunity to get away.

SKILLS IN CONTEXT 1

ATTEMPTED GRAB

Intercepting an attack early places you in a stronger position

The earlier we can intervene, the better our chances of success. In this case Lena recognizes the intent to grab her as the attacker approaches her. She has her hands up and is ready to react appropriately before he can get his hands onto her.

By taking the inside position, Lena takes control of his neck immediately and pulls his head while she pushes her thumb into his eye. Her attack is so short and sudden that he will have difficulty reacting before it's too late.

As he tries to protect his eye, Lena quickly shifts gears and, seeing his hands come up to his face, kicks the groin. By successfully reading his body, she is able to take advantage of split-second opportunities such as these to prevent him from mounting any renewed attack. She throws several groin kicks, taking advantage of the time that each one buys her.

As he bends to protect his groin and react to the pain, Lena senses the opportunity to make her escape. She pushes his

Incoming Grab

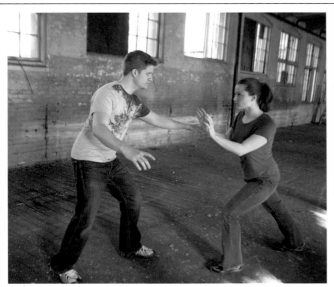

- In this example Lena's awareness is very good. She reads her assailant's body language and is prepared for action when he comes close.

- As he raises his arms to grab her, she brings her own arms to the inside, looking for the dominant, controlling position.

- She knows that she can better defend herself from the grab by establishing a strong clinch tie, so she is ready and in position before he makes contact.

Attack the Eye Immediately

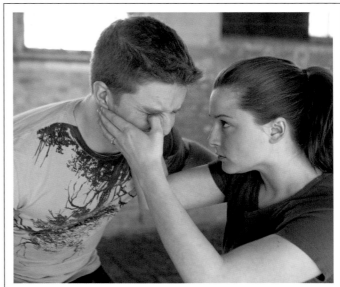

- Lena swims her arms into position at the neck and wastes no time in beginning her counterassault.

- As her first hand reaches the back of the neck, she digs the other thumb into the attacker's eye. She knows that this attack to a sensitive area can create a powerful reaction.

- There is no sense in waiting to be hit first. Because she properly assessed the aggression, she takes the initiative and does not yield it.

shoulders to make sure he is unable to grab her, and, with a big shove away, she turns to run.

Attack the Unprotected Groin

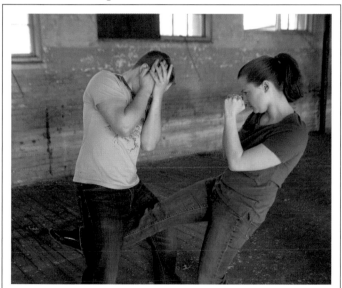

- As the attacker's hands go to protect his injured eye, Lena sees another opportunity arise.

- She transitions quickly to a groin kick as the hands commit to his face.

- Not only will he not have time to defend the kick, but also he will likely not even see it.

- Here Lena has taken the initial advantage and continued to press forward aggressively so that her attacker will not have time to respond.

Disengaging

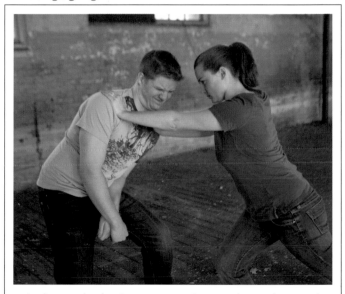

- As the attacker begins to respond to the groin kick, Lena sees an opportunity to make her escape.

- She has landed two significant attacks. Although they will not incapacitate her assailant for long, she will make the most of the time she has.

- Lena pushes on her attacker's shoulders to make sure she isn't grabbed on the way out. She shoves her attacker away and turns to run, while he is still realizing what has happened.

THE MOUNT POSITION
Take control of a bigger, stronger attacker

The mount position allows you to control your attacker by placing your weight on and around him effectively. You can use this position to neutralize upper-body strength and to tire and hold someone who is uncooperative.

The key element to pinning from the mount is the control it provides over your attacker's hips. By hooking your lower legs around his hips and supporting our weight in our arms, you can create a position that forces him to struggle against your weight in order to move. Although the position has specific characteristics, it's important to stay flexible in their application. If an attacker tries to roll you off him, it may be necessary to stick a hand or a foot out for balance in order to avoid falling. This is not only acceptable but also encouraged. Preserve your advantageous position by remaining open to adjustment as necessary.

The mount is not only a position of control but also one

Controlling the Mount

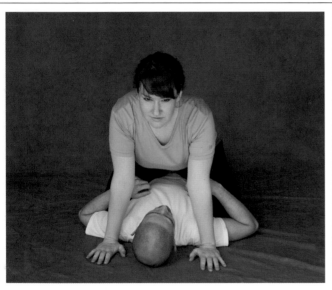

- In the mount position, you have an advantage over your attacker because you limit his movement.

- Keep your weight in your knees (and sometimes your hands) to trap him into a position where his avenues for escape are limited.

- Because gravity never tires, you can use your weight in this position in order to tire out someone who is struggling against you.

- Be flexible in this position. If you need to adjust your balance, do so.

Foot Position

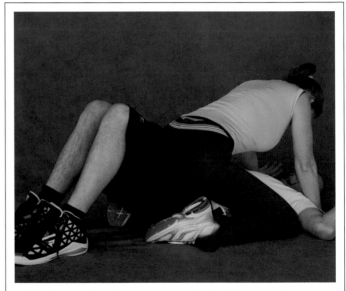

- The feature that gives the mount its strength is the position of the feet.

- Depending on your attacker's height and the length of your leg, you should hook your feet underneath the thigh, hips, or back.

- By hooking your feet, you create a pulling motion with your legs that glues your weight to your attacker. It forces him to struggle with your weight as he tries to move.

- If he tries to push you off, pull your feet toward your butt to make this difficult.

in which you can continue counterattacking with punches, slaps, attacks to the eyes, biting, and more. You can grab handfuls of dirt and throw them in his face. You can find an impromptu weapon and strike him with it. The mount is a tremendously advantageous place for you to be.

Using the Arms

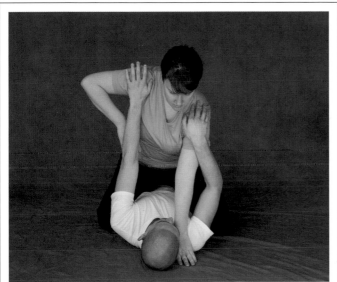

- It's common for people underneath the mount to push up on your chest and shoulders to try to escape.

- If this happens, sway and twist your upper body from side to side. Doing this makes it more difficult for him to establish a strong push against you.

- Also you can swim the arms inside his (and to the ground) to dislodge his hands. Replacing your hands on the ground also reestablishes your balance, which is important when someone tries to push you off.

Striking from the Mount

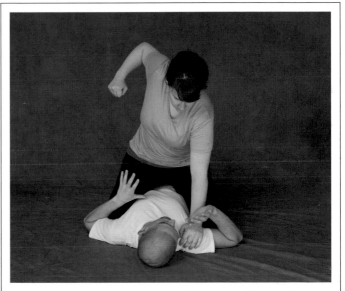

- Punches are the most common choice, rained down using one or both fists. You can also modify these into palm strikes to protect your hands or hammering strikes with the fist.

- You can strike with the elbows, using either the pointy tip of the elbow or the broad side of the forearm.

- When you are in mount, gravity aids your strikes. Throw as much weight into them as you can!

THE SIDE POSITION
Pin and immobilize someone in order to establish control

When it comes to pinning someone down, the holddowns from the side position reign supreme. These positions allow you to powerfully immobilize the attacker's weight and can be particularly difficult for him to escape.

The key elements to the holddowns from the side are pressure on his chest and the neutralization of his arms.

When you hold someone down from the side, you create tremendous friction by placing yourself chest to chest with

him. In particular, focus on the areas where the chest and shoulder come together because if he attempts to turn over, pressure on these areas will prevent him from doing so.

In order to maintain that pressure, anchor your weight to his upper body using your arms. Hugging and pulling motions under the shoulder and neck fasten your weight to his body, making him struggle against you (and your invisible friend, gravity).

Holding from the Side

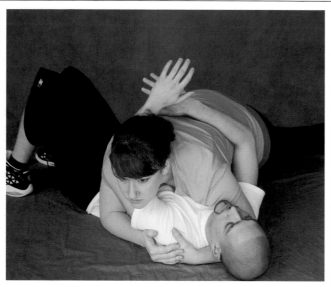

- When pinning from the side, place your weight chest to chest with your attacker.

- You primarily use your arms to attach yourself and your legs to balance.

- Place your chin on the collarbone or in the armpit

- to make it more difficult for the opponent to attack your head.

- Focus on applying your weight to the far side of the chest, where it meets the shoulder. This is a key component to keeping him flat on his back.

Arm Positioning

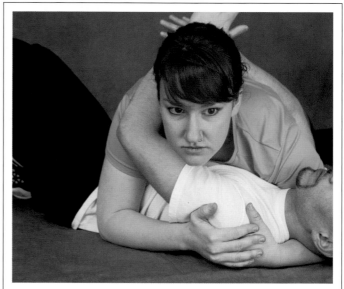

- In this holddown from the side, you establish two strong pulling motions with the arms.

- The most critical one is the arm under the neck—by pulling tightly with your forearm you make yourself feel very heavy.

- The other arm comes underneath the shoulder, like an underhook, and assists in pulling the shoulder to your chest.

- If you need to catch your balance, the arm under the shoulder is usually the preferred tool. You can use the hand or the elbow.

After you have established this position, make it difficult for him to use his arms to push you away. When you maintain close contact and strong pulls, he cannot simply bench press you off of himself. If you keep your hips low to the ground and your legs wide for balance, he will not be able to roll you over. By tucking your face against him, you make it difficult for him to push or strike it.

Leg Positioning

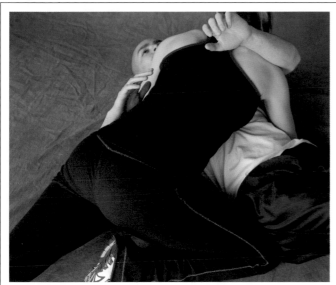

- Your knee closest to his legs will drive under his thigh or hip. This stops him from moving his legs toward or underneath you, limiting his ability to control your body.

- Your leg closest to his head is extended out like a pushup: knee off the ground, heel raised, and weight on the ball of the foot. This foot drives your weight forward into his chest if he tries to push you back.

- The hips are held very low to the ground to avoid being lifted and rolled over.

A Second Variation

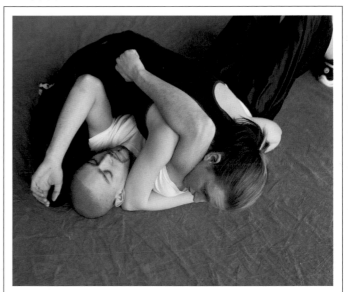

- In this variation of pinning from the side, the goal is to keep his arms in an awkward position; if they are stuck alongside his head, it is extremely difficult for him to push you away.

- Although this holddown doesn't have the strong pulling motion of the first one—the arm under his neck—it does create control by removing his options.

- Most untrained people will not be able to escape this pin without the use of their arms.

THE CLOSED GUARD
Use your legs to control an attacker at close range

If you find yourself on the bottom of a wrestling situation, you can still establish control by using your legs. This is a technique known as the "guard" position. The first variation we'll explore is the "closed" guard, in which your ankles are crossed behind your attacker's back.

This position is used for defensive purposes to hold onto your assailant and make it difficult for him to grab or strike you effectively. It limits his ability to move and allows you to

tie up his arms so that he cannot easily use them.

For women this is a particularly strong position because they are gifted with strength and dexterity in their hips that men are not. The closed guard turns this gift into a decided advantage because it translates this aptitude into the strength to hug and control by using the legs.

Using the arms in addition to the legs creates an added dimension of control and brings us to the true reason why

The Closed Guard

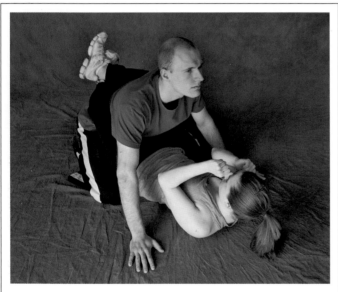

- To establish the closed guard, wrap your legs around your attacker's waist and cross your ankles.

- Doing this gives you the ability to use your strongest muscles—those of the hips and legs—to push, pull, and hold.

- Using your legs from underneath helps you neutralize a strength advantage. You can keep him off balance and put him in positions where it is difficult for him to do you harm.

Hugging the Head and Arm

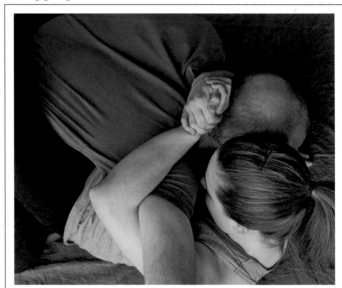

- With your closed guard established, one strong way to attach your upper body is to hug the head and one arm together.

- Bring your forearm against the back of the neck and swim your other hand under his arm like an under-hook. Clasp your hands

and squeeze his head and arm together with your forearms.

- If you can, turn his face into his bicep to make it more difficult for him to orient himself or recruit strength in his arm.

the closed guard is such a dominant position: The attacker on top is able to fight with only two arms, whereas the defender on bottom uses four limbs (two arms and two legs).

Climbing the Legs

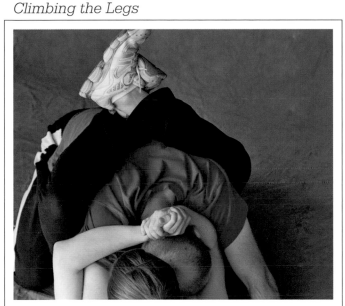

- If your attacker's upper body is close to you, increase your control by climbing your legs up high on his back.

- Doing this allows you to directly neutralize the strength of his upper body with your legs. It makes it difficult for him to move or to use his arms effectively.

- In this position you can sometimes free one or both of your own arms in order to strike.

Hanging from the Guard

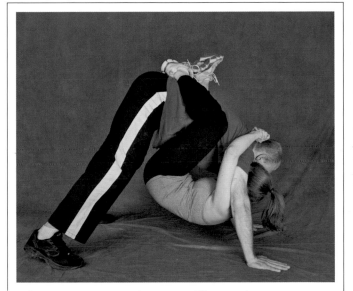

- In some cases an attacker will try to stand up or lift himself while trapped in your closed guard.

- You can tire him by hanging your weight off of his body, forcing him to carry both of you.

- If he stands up, you can release your legs and stand up, too. This can be your opportunity to push away and disengage.

- Be wary of the possibility that he will lift you from the ground only to slam you back down.

THE OPEN GUARD
Maintain distance to avoid being pinned to the ground

The open guard position is similar to the closed guard—you will use your legs to defend against an attacker who is trying to pin you to the ground. With the open guard, we do not cross our ankles around his back but instead use the feet and knees as part of a barrier between us.

The open guard is a tool for creating and maintaining distance between ourselves and our attacker. It keeps him at bay because it limits his ability to drive his weight forward and reach us. It pushes his weight back, so that he cannot pin us down. It keeps his head and shoulders away, so he cannot grab us.

The open guard is a valuable position because it preserves our ability to move easily. In this position you can scoot about on your hands, feet, and hips. You can avoid your assailant, and you can stand up quickly. Whereas the closed guard provides close-quarter defense, the open

The Open Guard

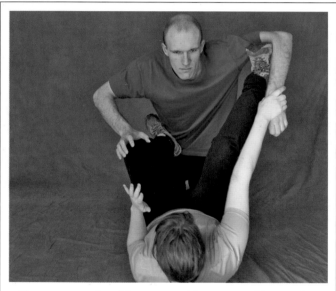

- The open guard position keeps distance between yourself and your attacker through the use of pushing motions.

- Rather than lying flat on your back, assume a mobile body position (sitting up or sitting on one hip).

- The more pushing motions you put on the front of his body, the better. They serve as obstacles that prevent him from moving forward to place his weight on top of you.

- Keep your hands, feet, elbows, and knees in between the two of you.

Feet on the Biceps

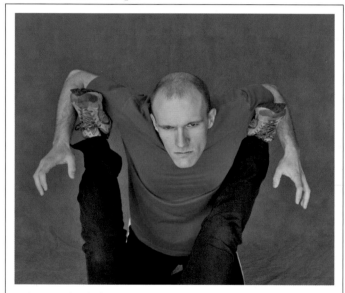

- One method of using the open guard is to directly engage his arms using your legs.

- Here you neutralize his arms by placing a stronger tool—your legs—against them.

- Grasp his wrists and place

the edge of each foot inside the crook of his elbow. Pull on his hands as you push with your feet.

- Because most men depend on the strength of their upper body, this method can help you to even the playing field if he is bigger or stronger.

guard provides medium-range freedom.

You can use the open guard both as a progression from the closed guard and as the failsafe before it. If someone has pushed you to the ground and is trying to hold you there, you can stop him from closing the distance by using the pushing tools of the open guard. If you fail to keep him back, the closed guard will be your next stop.

Similar to the closed guard, the open guard is especially advantageous for women. It turns hip strength and dexterity into a concrete advantage that you can pit against upper-body strength. The open guard allows you the same four limbs-versus-two limbs advantage that the closed guard provided plus the freedom to move.

Pushing Tools and Targets

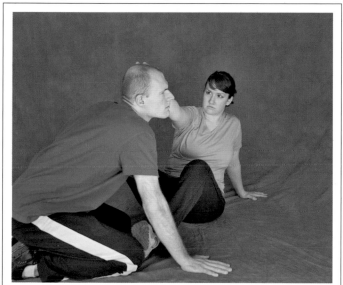

- When you push, the best targets for your pushes are the biceps, hips, knees, and head.

- The hips are the most important because they house his center of gravity. Keep distance between his weight and your body.

- Keeping his head at a distance makes it harder for him to grab or strike with his arms.

- Pushing on his knees can stop him from following you or can topple him off balance.

Hooking Tools

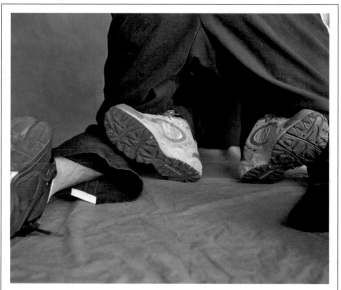

- When an attacker tries to move around your pushing tools, you can incorporate a second set of skills: hooking motions.

- By hooking a foot behind his knee, you make it difficult for him to flank you. He cannot move to the side without bringing you along.

- Hooking under the legs also allows you to off-balance your attacker by lifting him up. The hooked feet give you access to his center of gravity from underneath.

HEADLOCKS

Untrained attackers commonly try to grab the head for control

Headlocks are a choice attack of the untrained wrestler. For some primal reason, the visceral reaction of most untrained fighters is to target the head. If they're trying to box, they aim punches at the head. If they're trying to wrestle, they grab the head and squeeze.

Headlocks can be a particularly uncomfortable experience, whether applied standing or on the ground. The pressure on the head and neck can be painful, and the headlock can be

used as an opportunity to throw punches at the face.

If you find yourself in a headlock while standing, your main priority should be to escape without going to the ground. Establish your balance and immediately attack your assailant in order to break free. Of course, you can prevent the headlock by establishing good position in the clinch and controlling his arms.

If you're on the ground when the headlock is applied, you

Headlock on the Ground

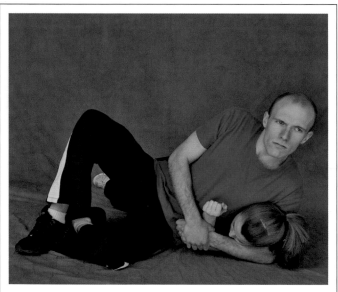

- Wrestlers are commonly taught the headlock as a common means of throwing and pinning someone, though many other grappling styles do not use it or use it sparingly.

- If someone has a significant strength, size, or weight advantage, this will be a difficult situation to escape.

- When stuck in a headlock, it's important that you turn onto your side to face your attacker and tuck your chin. Doing this helps reduce the pressure on your neck and the risk of a choke.

Headlock Dangers

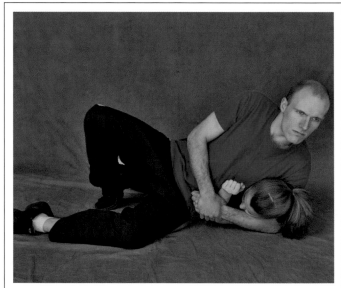

- Headlocks are not often chokes—that is, they do not put pressure directly onto the windpipe or the blood pathways that supply the brain.

- It can be difficult to breathe, however, because of the other person's weight on your chest.

- A headlock can also put tremendous strain on the neck to the point of causing a serious injury.

- On top of that, a headlock can simply be incredibly painful because of the pressure on the chest and neck.

must do your best to turn onto your side and create space. Failing that, you can take advantage of the opportunities to attack his eyes and bite his forearm or the side of his body.

Although the headlock is rarely a significant threat in and of itself, it presents danger by limiting your ability to defend yourself and to escape.

Headlock When Standing

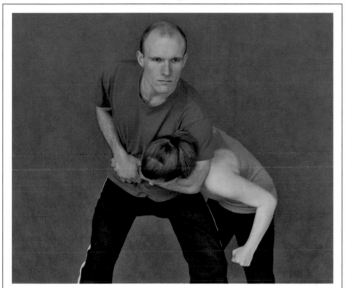

- Headlocks commonly start standing up, in the clinch range. Many untrained attackers will try to grab the head out of desperation.

- The headlock itself is not particularly dangerous, but the position makes it tough to defend yourself

against punches from the free hand.

- Also, if you are pulled off balance with the headlock, you can be taken to the ground in this position. This will be a much worse situation, and there is a risk of injury as you fall.

Head and Arm Control

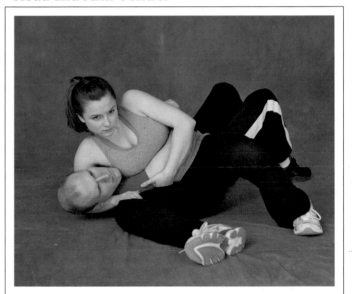

- Almost every grappling system incorporates some kind of "head and arm" control position for pinning.

- Called "*kesa gatame*" (meaning "scarf hold") in Japanese judo and jujitsu, this method of pinning is extremely difficult to escape.

- It also has advantages that a simple headlock does not, like its ability to keep one's attacker flat on the ground.

- Although we do not typically encourage the use of headlocks as a method of control, a head and arm position can be a tremendously effective tool.

STANDING & DOWN
How to handle a hostile approach when you are seated

To be approached by someone while you are seated can be an intimidating encounter. You find yourself at a disadvantage, and it can be difficult to get away if the interaction turns heated. Our approach to this situation is to remain calm and to establish a position, however unassuming, that removes some elements of our disadvantage.

Prop yourself up on one arm and turn so that you are not facing your aggressor directly but rather at a slight profile.

Minimize the amount of your body that is exposed to him as a target while supporting yourself in the direction facing him. Keep your head away from him and use your free arm as a barrier if necessary.

By placing yourself in a mobile, supported position, you can easily turn to face someone who tries to reach you with grabs or strikes. You make it difficult for him to flank you, which is immensely valuable in any kind of wrestling situation. If all

Sitting versus Standing

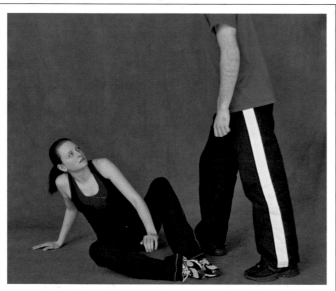

- If you are caught unaware, you may need to defend yourself against someone standing over you.

- The disadvantages of this position are great: It is hard for you to strike with power or to escape a wrestling match.

- Because you are already on the ground, you are that much closer to being pinned there.

- You must act quickly in this position to avoid missing your window of opportunity—whether your decision is to escape or to engage.

Legs between the Two of You

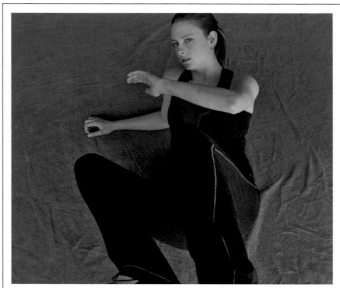

- The most important tool that can keep your assailant away from you is your legs.

- The legs can be used to maintain distance between the two of you, making it difficult for him to hit or grab you.

- You can also push with the legs to make sure he cannot drive his weight on top of your body.

- By keeping the legs tucked in, you can also be ready to kick at any opportunity.

else fails and he tries to grab you, you can easily begin using the open guard for control.

Most importantly, being upright and mobile will allow you to rise to your feet easily in order to put some distance between yourself and your attacker.

Defending with the Arms

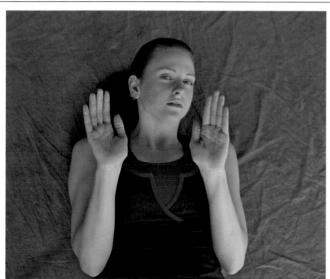

- Keep your hands in front of your face to help deflect any punches or attempts to grab your head.

- In this position you are also ready to push with your hands and elbows if your attacker tries to get close and is able to bypass your legs.

- Tuck your elbows to your ribs in order to defend against punches or kicks to your midsection.

- With your knees and elbows tucked, it is also more difficult for someone to pin you to the ground.

Propped Up and Mobile

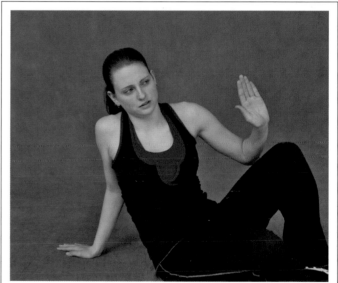

- It's important that you maintain your ability to move freely in the seated position. Lying flat on your back will inhibit you.

- Minimize the surface area (and resulting friction) between your body and the ground.

- Place your weight onto one hip and one hand, so that you can move lightly and easily.

- From here you can easily spin to face your attacker if he attempts to move around your arms and legs.

KICKING FROM OPEN GUARD
The benefit to being on your back is the ability to use your legs

Kicking is the most natural extension of the open guard. Because the legs are already engaged as pushing tools on the front of the attacker's body, it is a natural extension of the situation to begin striking with the feet.

The targets that may be available to you depend a bit on range. If he is standing up or is far away, you may be able to plant a solid heel in his groin. If he is closer, you may choose to kick him in the face instead. Wherever you aim, recover

quickly to maintain control. Strike a balance between kicking and pushing. If you kick too much, you may lose the control that the open guard affords with its pushing motions of the feet and knees. On the other hand, if you offer too little offense, your attacker will not suffer for trying to pin you down. Deliver sharp kicks, measured against the control you can preserve.

Keep him afraid of the damage you can cause with kicks in

Upkick to the Face

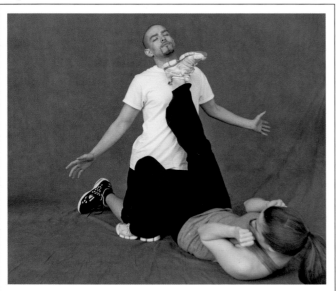

- One way to buy yourself time (and distance) is to drive the heel of your foot into your attacker's face.

- The action is similar to stomping your foot, and it uses the same strong muscle groups.

- Make contact with the nose, mouth, temple, eye, or the underside of the chin.

- Throw several quick, strong kicks to drive him off of you. Be sure to throw your hips into the kick for power.

Upkick to the Groin

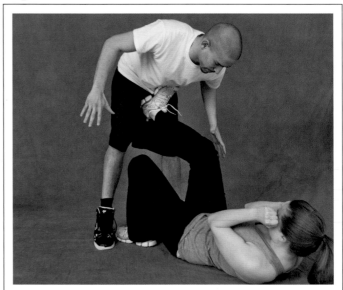

- Kicking the groin fulfills a couple of objectives when you're on your back:

- The pain it causes can discourage your attacker from continuing the assault or at least be a distraction that buys you time.

- Stomping at the groin in this way also pushes his hips backward, which can knock him off balance.

- Drive the heel of your shoe into the groin. The tougher or pointier the heel of the shoe, the better.

this position. A good impact to the face or groin should buy you the time to stand or perhaps even to run. And if the first kick doesn't succeed, keep firing them until one does.

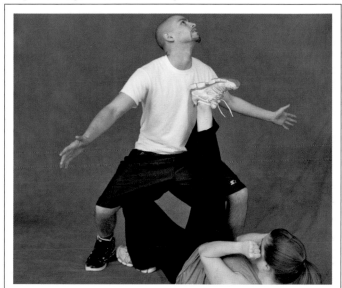

··········· GREEN ● LIGHT ···········

When kicking from the guard, coil your knees to your chest and then spring forward, driving your hips off of the ground and pushing your heel squarely into its target. Make use of the strong muscles of the leg, hip, and back, all in unison. Recoil after impact and recheck that you still have control. Then prepare to fire another kick.

Kick to the Thigh

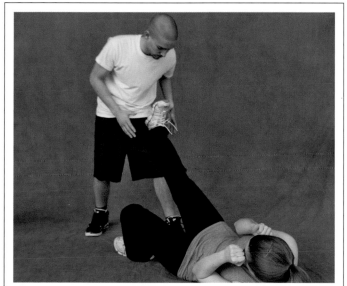

- When the distance between you and your assailant is greater, you can drive a heel downward into the thigh.

- Use a chopping motion as you kick down into the muscle of the thigh. This is a less invasive target than the groin.

- Although this kick lacks the space-preserving benefits of a pushing-style kick, it can still be an effective way to make your opponent back off, creating space for you to get to your feet.

Upkick against Standing Attacker

- If your attacker is standing over you, it is still possible to throw a kick to the face. Lift your hips into the air and drive your leg upward.

- A kick to the face here can take your attacker by surprise and is actually a powerful technique.

- Drive your feet into the face or under the chin.

- If you cannot reach the face, kick the groin first. If the groin kick lands solidly, it may bend him forward, bringing his head into range.

AVOIDING STRIKES FROM GUARD

Strikes thrown from above have gravity behind them, so defense is critical

Defending against strikes is an important aspect of controlling from the guard. By controlling the distance, you can take your attacker's biggest weapons away from him.

Pull him forward onto his hands by pulling your knees to your chest. If you can force him to place his weight in his hands, he cannot simultaneously be using them to punch.

Make him carry your weight as he tries to lift himself up. Entangle his arms so that it is difficult for him to pull himself away.

By keeping his upper body parallel to the ground, you force him to keep his hands on the ground or to lay his weight onto you. If he chooses to lie on you, swing your knees from

Deflecting Punches and Hits

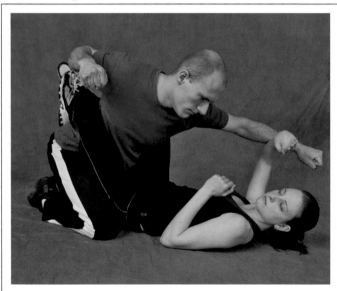

- The most common attack inside the guard is a punch or slap to the face.

- Deflect hits in this position by bringing your arms to the center. It will be easier to defend yourself here if you force the attacker to hit in wide, looping arcs.

- If you can, make contact at the bicep or inside of the elbow. You can prevent punches using bicep control, just as you did in the clinch range.

- Even if your blocking isn't perfect, it will be better than taking punches to your unprotected face.

Wrap the Upper Arm

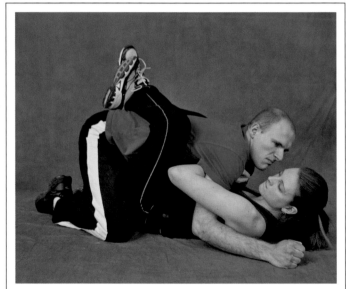

- Bring your attacker close to you by pulling him forward with your knees as he punches.

- If your arms are in the center, it will be easy to reach over the top of his arms as he catches his balance.

- Hug around the upper arm with your forearm. Doing this makes it difficult for him to pull the arm free and to grab or strike you.

side to side and rock him off balance. You may even be able to roll him over and establish the mount!

Most people will instinctively catch their balance in this position. When he does this, he cannot strike you. Take advantage of this position and initiate whatever offense you choose: bite him, hit him, drive your thumb into his eye. But first and foremost, take away his ability to hit you. With gravity on his side, you do not want to be exchanging strikes with someone on top of you!

Hugging the Head and Arm

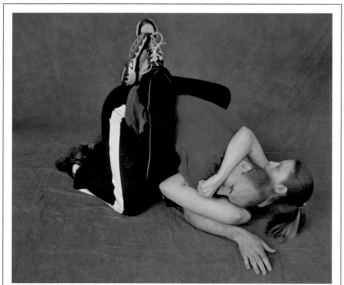

- After you have wrapped the arm, hug his head close to you.

- If he can't lift his head, he can't throw any big, strong punches.

- He also won't be able to free the arm you've wrapped because he can't pull his shoulders away from you.

- Continue pulling with your legs as you hold the head and arm tightly.

- Use your forearms to hold because they are stronger than your hands.

Blocking the Far Side

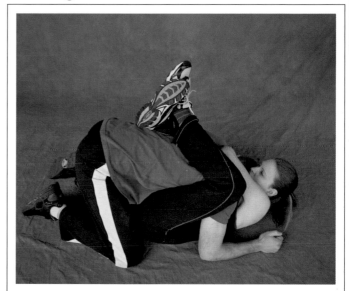

- Hugging the head and arm leaves one of his arms free. You need to address that arm, or else you'll take punches to the back or side of the face.

- On the side of his free arm, bring your leg up high on the back. Pinch your knee up to your elbow—the one that's hugging his head.

- By bringing your knee and elbow together, you're limiting the movement of his arm. This makes it tough for him to strike with it.

135

ATTACKING FROM CLOSED GUARD

Cause damage from your back while keeping your attacker under control

Facing an attacker in your closed guard position, you must create space in order to get away to safety. The primary tool for creating space here is intense pain.

When you latch onto him with the closed guard and entangle his arms so that he cannot strike you, you create what appears to be a stalemate position. Neither of you can take

the advantageous position to pin the other down, and he is unable to strike at you. From here you can launch quickly into some vicious and aggressive attacks, including biting and attacking his eyes. These attacks cause tremendous pain and threat of injury, and the most common response is to pull away—he will try to escape your attack.

Bite the Face

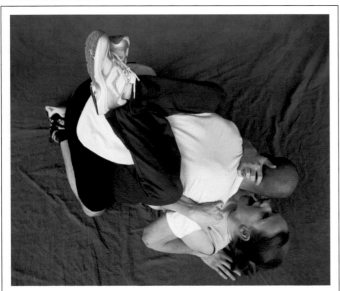

- The advantage of the closed guard is that you use the combined strength of your arms and legs to keep your attacker controlled.

- Because he has forced such close quarters, he has placed himself in a position where he cannot escape the bite.

- Hug the head and shoulders and bite the side of the neck, face, ear, and shoulder.

- The goal is to cause him to panic and to push away. If he moves away, you can get to your feet.

Thumb to the Eye

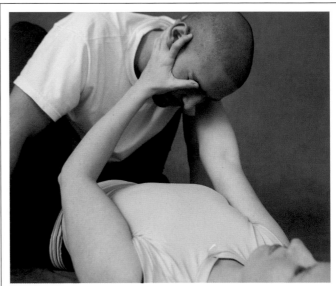

- With the head controlled, you can also use a thumb to the eye to create pain, injury, and panic.

- Hug the back of the head so he can't escape. Drive your thumb into his eye. Pull on his head to increase the power of your attack.

- Aim to cause intense pain and to impair vision, creating the distraction you need to stand up and get away.

If he lifts his weight away from you, that's good news. This will be your opportunity to let go and escape to standing. From there you can make your escape or reinitiate your attack in a much improved situation.

Be aggressive in your attacks from this position. You must overwhelm him with the urge to get away from you. If he doesn't feel threatened, he will try to smother you with his weight or find ways to strike at you. See the opportunities for attack before he does. Be vicious.

MAKE IT EASY

When you engage in close-quarter attacks such as biting and eye gouging, do so in positions where your attacker cannot do it right back to you. Here in the closed guard, with his arms entangled and supporting him on the ground, you can attack without fear that he will strike you or gouge at your eyes. Control his head when you bite, and you can remove the fear of mutual biting as well.

Elbow to the Head

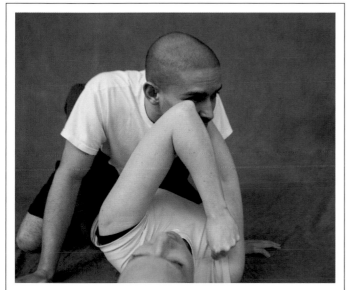

- If the distance is a bit greater, you can strike with the elbow from the closed guard.

- Hold the head with one hand and deliver strikes with the tip of the elbow. At this range you can hit the eye, nose, and temple.

- Elbow strikes can cause cuts or damage the small bones of the face because the small surface area creates tremendous pressure on impact.

- Strike viciously and repeatedly with the elbow while pulling him into the strikes.

Punching from Guard

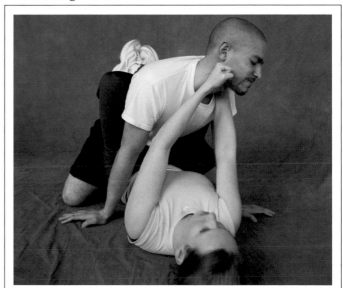

- If he is too far away to bite, thumb, or elbow, consider punching from your back.

- Gravity puts you at a disadvantage, and your body position on your back makes it hard to punch with full power.

- Hold the head and pull him into the strikes to improve their effect. Throw many strong, fast punches.

- Although the punches from here will not end a fight, they can create the opportunity to push him away and get to your feet.

ATTACKING UNDER THE SIDE
Causing pain and injury can help you create the space to escape if you're pinned down

Underneath the side you are in a position of great disadvantage. It's critical that you attack your assailant immediately in order to create the opportunity to move and escape.

Although being held from the side is a tough position to escape, it carries few particular threats. In general it is more of a situation in which you are likely to feel pinned as opposed

to a situation in which you are worried about being struck or choked. When placed here by someone much bigger or heavier, you can feel crushed, as though it is difficult to move or breathe, so you must attack him to regain the freedom to move.

Your goal in attacking him is to create space. Specifically,

Bite the Body

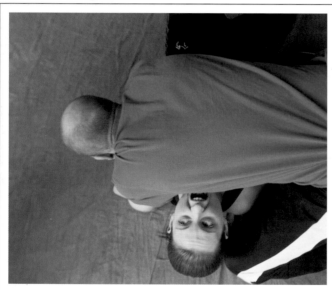

- When you are trapped under the side, the side of the body is often within reach of your teeth.

- Bite sensitive areas such as the nipple or the latissimus dorsi ("lat") muscle, which forms the back of the armpit.

- Use many quick, sharp bites. Do not try for a whole mouthful.

- If possible, hug his body, so that he cannot pull away easily. Doing this will cause him to try a lot harder to get away from you.

Knee to the Head

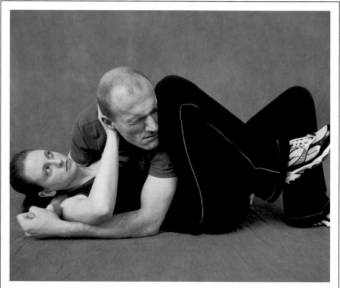

- With his head to the side of your body, you can sometimes clear a path to strike his head with a knee.

- Push his head into the path of the knee with your hand and bring the knee up swiftly and forcefully.

- Aim for the back of his head and neck. Alternatively, you can hit the side of the head or the face if he turns his head.

you must force him to take his weight off of your chest. After he has done that, you can immediately turn onto your side, push yourself up onto a hand or elbow, and get up off of your back.

Given even a tiny bit of space, you can push him away and try to bring your legs in between the two of you for the open or closed guard positions. Having successfully arrived there, you can further assess the situation and look for the opportunity to stand up and to escape.

········· GREEN ● LIGHT ·············

The best attacks in a situation such as this one are the ones that will cause him to pull away from you instinctively. For this reason gouging the eye and biting are two primary strategies because they will cause him not only to release you with his arms but also to take his body off of you in an attempt to flee your attack as it continues.

Thumb to the Eye

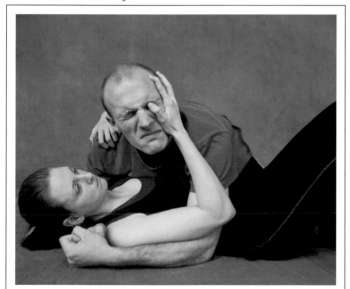

- Underneath the side it's common for his head to be near your shoulder. If your hand is free, drive your thumb into the eye.

- If possible, hold his head with your free hand. This may not be an option, depending on the position of his body as he tries to pin you down.

- Thumb the eye to create distraction and to motivate him to take his weight off of your chest.

- Removing his weight from your chest is the number one factor in escaping from underneath the side.

Grab the Groin

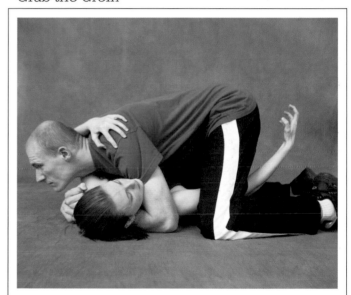

- When underneath the side, sometimes you find that your arm is trapped under your attacker's leg.

- Having your arm pinned makes it difficult to defend yourself against punches, slaps, grabs, or chokes. It can also make it tricky to hold onto him when biting, thumbing, or kneeing.

- If you find your arm beneath him, take advantage of the situation and grab the groin.

- A successful groin attack here can lift his weight from your body as he tries to avoid your grab.

ATTACKING UNDER THE MOUNT
In vulnerable positions you must act quickly and aggressively

Being under the mount is an extremely dangerous situation. Here you are vulnerable to punches and chokes that will have your attacker's full weight behind them. For this reason it is crucial that you act as quickly as possible and aggressively.

The first objective is to protect your face and neck, which you can accomplish by hugging around his torso and burying your face against him. Pull tightly with your arms to make it hard for him to dislodge you in this position.

If he is low enough for you to reach his shoulders, an even better way to protect yourself is to hug him with one arm over his shoulders and one arm underneath. Pull him close to you with your arms in this position and bury your face against him. This will commit his weight to his arms because he must hold himself up. If he tries to sit up, he must carry your weight as well, which will require him to use his hands for balance. All this means that his hands are not available

Bite the Nipple

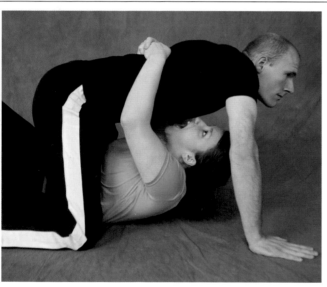

- As your assailant holds the mount position, hug your arms around his back tightly.

- Bring him close to you and bite the chest. Aim for the nipple.

- Bury your face against him as you bite. This protects you from being hit or punched and makes it difficult for him to escape your teeth; his best option should be to give up on the mount position entirely.

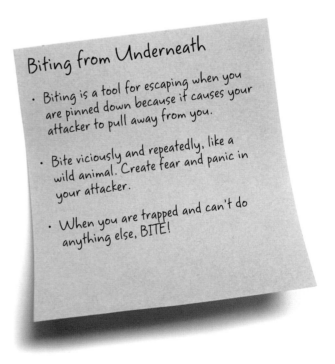

Biting from Underneath

- Biting is a tool for escaping when you are pinned down because it causes your attacker to pull away from you.

- Bite viciously and repeatedly, like a wild animal. Create fear and panic in your attacker.

- When you are trapped and can't do anything else, BITE!

to hit or choke you. After you have established some safety, begin your attack. Do not wait long because you are particularly vulnerable here.

• • • • • • • • • • • • • • • RED ● LIGHT • • • • • • • • • • • • • • •

If he is able to sit up in this position, this is a red alert situation: Punches are imminent! Dig your heels into the ground and drive your hips high into a bridge to destabilize his balance. As he falls forward, immediately hug around his upper body to prevent him from sitting up again.

Bite the Face

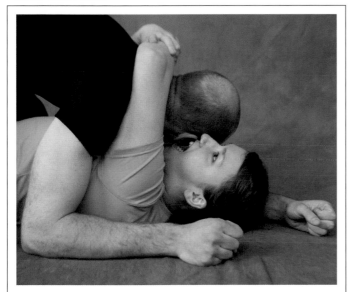

- One of the safest ways to control your attacker from underneath the mount is to wrap one arm over his shoulders and one arm under his armpit.

- Connect your hands or grab your own wrist to hug tightly in this position.

- With one arm over and one under, you can keep him very close to you. This situation minimizes the risk of being hit and puts you in a position to bite the ear or side of the face.

Thumb the Eye

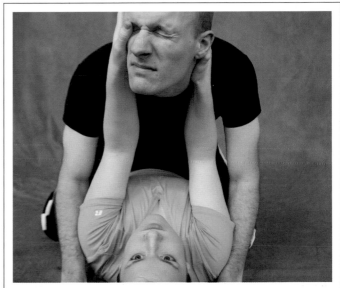

- If you can't reach with a bite, grab your attacker by the neck with one hand and thumb the eye with the other.

- Use the hand on the neck to make it difficult for him to get his head away from you.

- If he tries to lean back away from you, and you lose the ability to reach his face, hug around his torso and return to biting the chest.

ATTACKING INSIDE THE GUARD

If you find yourself controlled while on top, you can attack to create space and stand

It may come to pass that you find yourself on the top of the guard position and that you need to attack in order to neutralize the attack or to flee to safety. Take advantage of gravity's assistance as you rain down strikes from this position.

As you establish yourself here, you must be careful that your balance is not compromised. Create a wide base with your knees and sit with your hips low over your feet. If he pulls you forward, catch your balance by bracing your arms against the front of his body.

Many strikes are available to you in this position. The ones that will bring you the greatest result are always the attacks to the eyes, throat, and groin. Take advantage of the ability

Attack the Face

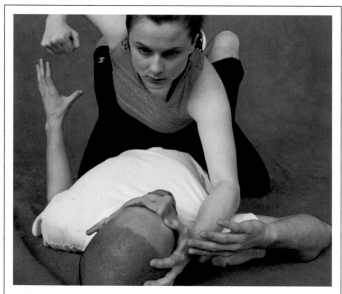

- Here are multiple objectives achieved simultaneously: While you hold his head down, you may be able to drive a thumb into his eye.

- At the same time you can punch or strike at his face using your fist like a hammer.

- When you're on top, you have a major advantage: gravity. Use it to its fullest potential by throwing your weight down into strikes.

- If you can pin his head, drive your weight into punches or hammering blows.

Knee to the Groin

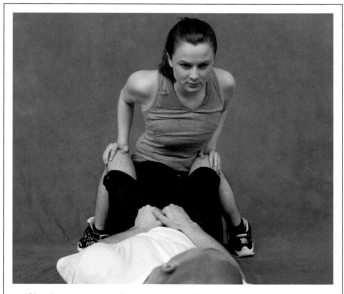

- If his legs open, and you can move, drive a knee down on top of his groin.

- The pain will make it difficult for him to use his legs effectively to control you. Use the opportunity to strike more or to escape the situation.

- Don't place your balance into the knee: He may try to roll over to protect himself from further injury.

- You can also use the knee to set up opportunities to throw strikes with your upper body.

to punch, hammer, and knee him with gravity's aid; it multiplies the force you put into your strikes if you can throw your weight downward into each one.

If you are able to stand, do so. Be wary of bringing your face close enough to him that he can grab, punch, or kick it. If you have created the distance to stand, you may have the opportunity to run, although it could require a few additional strikes to slow him down before you make your exit.

ZOOM

If you are stuck inside the closed guard and cannot get him to uncross his ankles and release you, punch the groin repeatedly. If the way in which your body types match up makes it difficult to do this effectively, stand up on both feet. This will stretch his position and make it much easier for you to punch the groin. Do so quickly and repeatedly to make him uncross his ankles.

Drive Forward and Bite

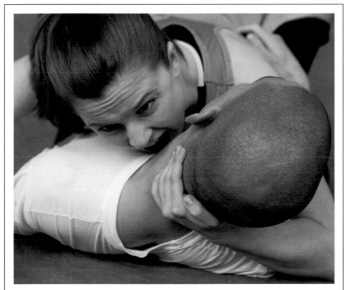

- If your attacker is holding you tightly, and you can't create the space to punch with the knee, drive forward into him.

- Place your shoulder onto his face, chin, or neck. Drive your weight into the shoulder and balance on your elbows.

- Bite the side of the face and neck. Do as much damage as possible until he tries to push you away with his arms. When he pushes, let go and back away.

Punch the Groin

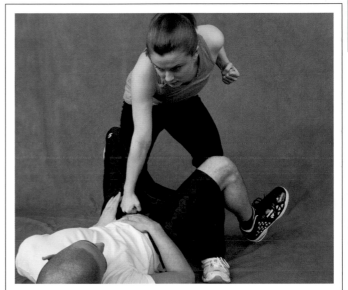

- If you can find the balance, stand up inside the guard position.

- Throw fast, repeated punches to his groin from here. Be aggressive.

- Because of the distance, it's difficult for him to grab your head or hit you when you stand, so you can let those fists fly.

- Be cautious of his ability to kick you in the face or groin in this position.

STANDING UP IN BASE
This safe way to stand under stress maintains balance and defense

Standing up "in base" is a smooth and natural way of moving from a seated position to a standing position. It allows you to protect your head with one arm during the entire maneuver, and it has extremely strong balance from front to back. If you find yourself threatened and need to stand, it is a safe way to do so.

The strength of this position comes from the fact that your body is always supported from behind. As you initiate, the supporting structure is your arm. As you lift your body, you place the leg in the same position, then remove the arm from the ground. There is no time when you are not fully braced from behind. Because of this, if an aggressor tries to push you back down as you stand, he will not be able to off-balance you. This method of standing is a natural one, though it is identified and practiced heavily in Brazilian Jiu-Jitsu training, where it is valued for its stability and protection.

Position Your Body

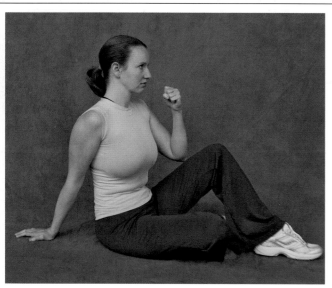

- In order to stand in base, position yourself on one hip.

- Support yourself on one hand and place it as close to your hips as you can comfortably.

- Bring your opposite foot close to your body, placing the heel into the ground.

- Your free hand can protect you during the process of standing if necessary.

- Relax the free leg and let it lie open. The position appears casual and should feel natural.

Lift Your Body

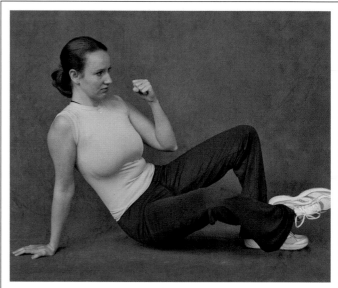

- Place your weight into the opposite hand and foot and lift your hips off of the ground.

- Although it may feel unusual to hold yourself up on one hand and one foot, with a little practice you can balance in this position easily.

- When kids do the "crab walk," they balance in this way, using opposite sides.

- Practice this on both sides of your body.

Be sure to support yourself on a flat palm and not on your hand perched up on the thumb and fingers. With your weight in the hand, a lifted palm can actually cause the thumb to dislocate. Flatten the palm to the ground to keep your joints safe.

MAKE IT EASY

Watch children stand up and sit down. Many of them use a method similar to this one naturally. It is a sensible and balanced way to stand. With some practice, it can actually become such a smooth set of movements that it can be done in less than a second. A movement that takes you from seated to standing in such a short amount of time is extremely valuable for self-defense situations.

Bring the Leg Underneath

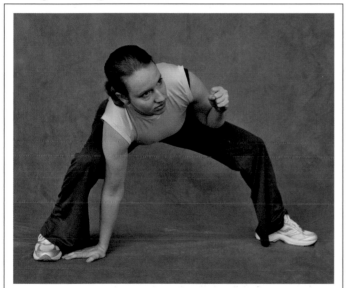

- After you have lifted your body, you can swing the free leg underneath you.

- Swing it deeply through the arch created by the arm and leg holding you up.

- Your free leg is going to replace the arm that's sup-porting you, but it needs to go all the way around it.

- When practicing, it helps to try to step on your own fingers.

- Don't let the knee touch the ground first!

Stand Up

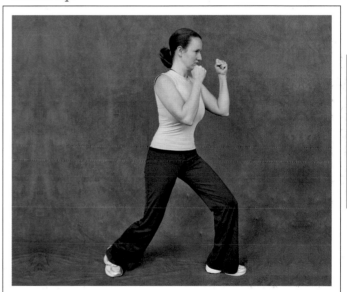

- After you place the foot on the ground, you can remove your hand and stand up.

- This method of standing up puts you into a strong stance. In particular you are quite stable from the front and back.

- You will find that you automatically have one side forward and that your free arm is already up to protect you.

- Practice this until you can do it quickly and smoothly.

KICKING TO STANDING

When threatened, you can use a kick to create the time to stand safely

Although standing up in base appears passive and unassuming, you can use it as a tool for a more aggressive way to get to your feet by adding a kick. Although most folks would naturally try to kick with the top leg, you need to make use of that leg for balance as you stand. Instead, you'll deliver a kick with the bottom leg, which is surprisingly powerful.

The key to the kick is that it develops unexpectedly. You appear to be sitting casually, and within a fraction of a second you are lifted and kicking.

As the leg retracts from the kick, it blends right into your motion of standing back up. Let the hips come backward from the kick and swing them directly into place to stand. By

Lift Your Body

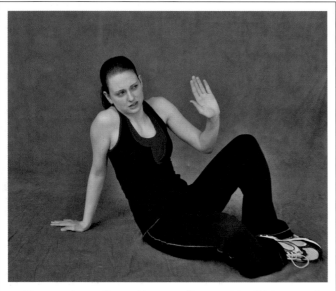

- When you're confronted by a standing assailant while sitting down, place yourself into the position to stand up in base.

- Protect your head with one arm and place your opposite hand and foot close by.

- Because it's a fairly natural way to sit, this all can be done nonchalantly to avoid raising suspicion before you strike.

- Lift your body up while keeping yourself balanced and protected.

Kick the Knee

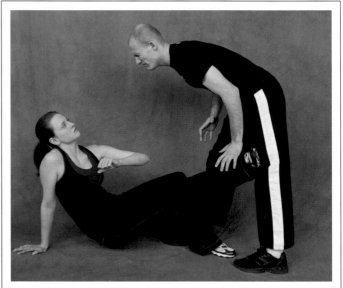

- With your weight lifted, you can throw a powerful kick with your free leg.

- Using your supporting arm and leg, swing your body forward to put your weight into the kick.

- Make contact with the bottom of your foot. You can turn it outward and strike with the entire sole or with the heel.

- Drive the foot into his shin or knee. If the groin is within range, kick it.

this method you can be on your feet and ready to continue as your aggressor is still reacting to the impact of the kick—which is exactly what we're after.

The kick can be used when you need to create the time or distance to stand—if he is too close to you, and you are concerned he will attack while you rise, use the kick to buy yourself the window of opportunity you need.

Prepare to Stand

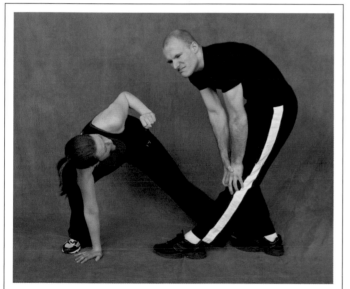

- After your kick makes contact, you will have a short opportunity to stand up if you act quickly.

- Immediately retract the kick and swing the leg underneath you in one smooth motion.

- Place the foot onto the ground in front of your hand. The sooner it lands there, the sooner you can stand up and continue fighting.

- Be sure to keep your eyes on your attacker while you're doing this. Practice standing up in base until you don't need to look.

Stand Up in Base

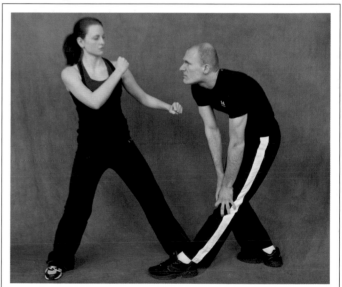

- With your balance maintained, come up into your stance.

- From start to finish, you must be able to do this entire series of movements, including the kick, in two seconds or less.

- During the entire transition, protect your head with your free hand and maintain eye contact on your assailant.

- From here you can move in and continue fighting back, or if you judge it possible, you can make your escape. If he comes at you again, you are in a much better position to defend yourself.

147

OPEN GUARD TO STANDING
Use your legs to push and create space to allow you to stand

The open guard position blends naturally with the opportunity to stand up from the ground. Because of its use of pushing tools and its goal of creating space, it presents numerous opportunities to push away from the attacker and quickly stand.

Using the open guard should be your primary defensive strategy when you are caught on your back. It is a position that will enable you to move, to hit, and to stand. If the open guard is insufficient, and your attacker is able to overwhelm your pushing motions, you can always fall back to the closed guard as a fail-safe and then work to reestablish the open guard. Similarly, if you find yourself trapped in a bad position such as the mount, the side, or a headlock, the open guard should be your immediate destination with the larger goal of creating the space to stand and open distance.

More than anything else, keep your attacker's weight off of

Pushing Tools

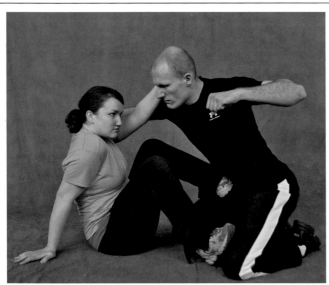

- The key to fighting from your back is to use every pushing tool at your disposal.

- Push him with your hands, elbows, feet, knees, and anything else that presents itself. Keep his head and hips away from you.

- If you can prevent him from pushing you all the way onto your back, this is ideal. It's much easier to stand from this position.

- If you are pushed all the way down, you will need to fight your way back to the open guard position in order to stand up easily.

Push the Chest

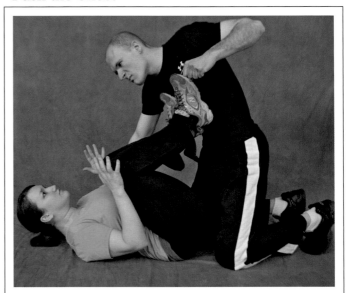

- If you are pushed all the way down, use your legs to keep him off of you.

- Push against his chest or hips with both feet. Doing this will keep him from throwing his weight down onto your upper body.

- Sometimes you can push him away explosively and buy yourself the time to stand all the way up.

- Women carry much of their strength in their hips and legs. Take advantage of this fact to neutralize his weight!

you in order to stand up. If he is able to come close enough that he can grab onto your body, especially around the midsection or upper body, it will be difficult to create space. Keep him away with your pushing tools in preparation to stand.

ZOOM

Open guard and its pushing motions are the primary tools for standing up since they focus on creating and defending space. With room between you and your attacker, you can stand up and make your exit, but if you can't create sufficient clearance, he will be able to pull you back down. Push him with your hands, elbows, knees, and feet so that he cannot stop you from getting to your feet.

Pinch the Knees

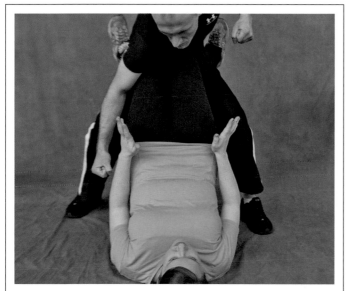

- If he gets by your feet and tries to hit or pin you, you can keep him away with your knees.

- Pinch them together and raise your hips up high. Doing this keeps him away from your face, so it's hard to strike or choke you.

- Pushing like this is strong, but it's hard to maintain for long. Push him away and quickly get to your feet.

- If you don't have time to stand, push with your knees and then push again using the soles of your feet.

Separate and Stand

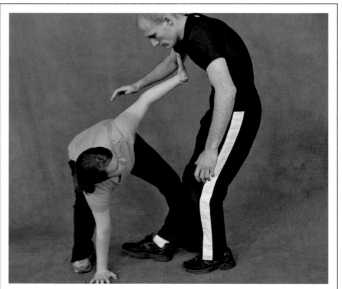

- After you establish strong pushes, give your attacker a big shove with your legs and stand up.

- The transition to standing from the open guard should be a quick one, provided you've been practicing standing up in base.

- The trick will be to buy yourself enough time to stand. Push him away with an explosive action. It may even knock him over!

- After you reach your feet, you can stand and fight or turn and run.

CLOSED GUARD TO STANDING

Even when you're in close quarters, you can push away with the legs

The closed guard is a difficult place to begin the process of standing because your attacker's weight is over (or even on top of) the trunk of your body. In order to disengage from him and make room to escape, you must create space where initially there is very little.

The safest way to begin the process is by entangling his arms and shoulders with your own. Hug him close to you and place the soles of both feet on his hips. You may need to place them one at a time, or if you have good dexterity and flexibility, you might be able to place both simultaneously.

As you release your grip with your arms, give a strong push with both legs. Slide yourself away from him. If his balance is

Control from Closed Guard

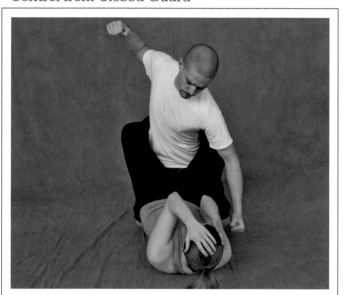

- The closed guard position is often used for extremely close quarters. The priority here is to make it difficult for him to lay his body weight on top of you.

- It can be difficult to separate from him if he can establish a strong hold on

you. Fight to control his arms if he tries to grab you.

- Although it sounds counterintuitive, it's easier to escape if he's trying to hit you—he's not holding on to your body, so you can push him away.

Feet on His Hips

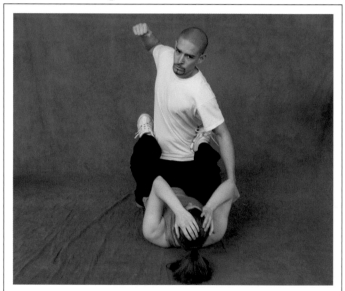

- When you feel the opportunity, place the soles of your feet onto his hips. You can do this one leg at a time or both at once.

- Bring your knees into the space between the two of you—they can help you defend if he's trying to strike you.

- Coil your body like a spring. You're going to push him away with all of your might.

- If he falls, stand up right away. If he is able to pursue you, use this to transition to open guard and continue pushing him away.

weak, this might actually slide him backward and away from you instead. With space established, quickly use the pushing tools from the open guard to keep him back as you begin the process of standing.

If he sits up, making it difficult for you to tie up his arms from the closed guard, you will need to push away from him quickly to avoid being hit with punches. You will have the advantage, though, of not fighting against the strength of his arms.

Push to Open Guard

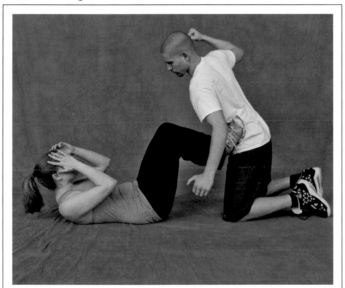

- Continue pushing him back using your hands and feet. Keep your knees between yourself and him and protect yourself with your hands.

- Defend the space between yourself and him. It will be difficult to get away if he can lay his weight onto you and even more so if he can establish a good grip on your body.

- By pushing him away from closed guard to open guard, you are widening the gap between the two of you. Soon you will have the opportunity to stand up.

Push Away and Stand

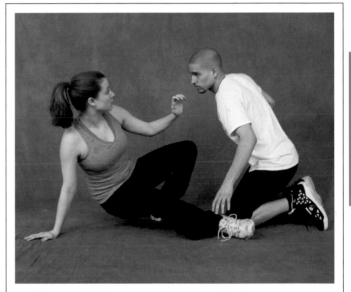

- When you feel the opportunity to push him back, drive him off with both legs and stand up in base.

- By moving from closed guard to open guard, you bring your pushing tools into play. Use those tools to create space and defend your freedom to move away.

- The most important asset is space. You won't get away without it, so push, push, push!

151

GRABBED FROM YOUR KNEES

Sometimes an attacker will attempt to tackle you as you try to stand

One of the most crucial moments in your escape to standing is the point when you disengage from your opponent and begin to rise. If you are kneeling or in the process of standing, he may try to grab around your body or legs in order to tackle you back to the ground.

The most critical skill in this situation is the ability to maintain your balance. By driving your feet as wide as possible, you can make it difficult for him to topple you. Focus on making

it as difficult as possible for him to surround your knees with his arms. Pry them apart with the muscles in your hips. Drive them to their maximum because he may try squeezing with both arms to bring them together.

The second priority is to make him struggle with your weight. Ideally, you want to place your center of gravity close to the ground, making it harder for him to lift you. Sag your hips down, driving the weight either in front of him or onto

Grabbed around the Legs

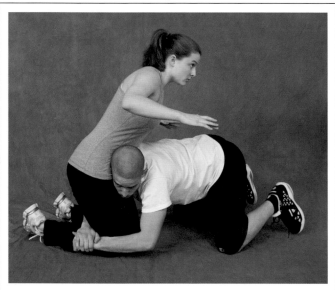

- Sometimes as you attempt to stand, your assailant may try to keep you from getting away by grabbing onto you.

- If your attacker grabs you around your legs, you must work hard to defend your balance and not be thrown onto your back.

- If your knees come together, it will be extremely difficult for you to stay upright. Do not allow him to hug them together.

Drive Your Hips Forward

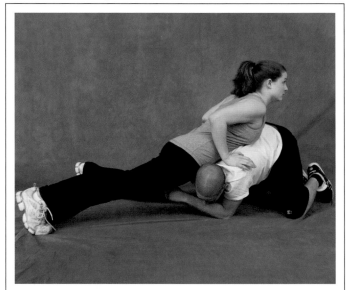

- Your first response must be to drive your hips forward and your weight down. Arch your back and push into him, so that he cannot tackle you backward.

- Spread your legs as far back and apart as you can. Doing this makes it difficult for him to collect them

together and compromise your balance.

- Create a wide base so that you cannot be rolled over. Make him struggle with carrying your weight while preventing him from holding both legs at once.

the back of his head. Arch your back to increase the force downward. Visualize driving his head into the ground using your bellybutton. You must fully apply your weight into this position to keep him from lifting you up.

Lastly, separate yourself from his upper body by peeling his head away. Try wedging both hands onto one of his ears and turning it awkwardly away from you. The farther his head moves, the less he can reach around you with his arms, so drive it as far as possible. Diminish his ability to pull and hold by taking his upper body off course. Having freed yourself

from his grip, move your body away and stand up. It's important that you maintain control of his head as you move away, in order to stop him from renewing his efforts to take you back to the ground.

Push the Head Away

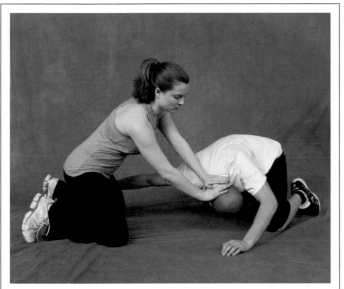

- As you continue defending your balance, make it even harder for him to grab your legs by pushing his head away.

- Wedge both hands against his head and push him off as hard as you can.

- Your goal is to separate his head and shoulders from your hips and legs so that he cannot hold them.

- Without a good grip, he cannot control your legs. By keeping his head away, you deny him a strong grab.

Stand and Separate

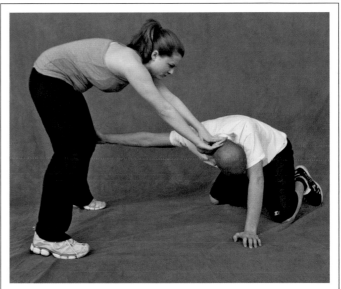

- As you peel his head off of you, come up to standing position. In this way you can continue making progress in your escape while shutting down his attack.

- Be sure to keep his head away from you so that he cannot chase your legs.

- If necessary, hold his head down while you deliver some kicks. Be careful not to allow him to grab your legs.

GRABBED WHILE STANDING

Some persistent attackers will grab around the legs when you are standing up

Sometimes an attacker is able to grab around your waist or legs. This can occur when you are in the clinch range or when you're almost finished standing up from the ground. This is a dangerous time, and you need to approach it carefully.

Your balance is critical. Broaden your base and do not allow your knees to come near each other. Sink your hips heavily

and arch your back. Push his head away to release yourself from his arms.

The danger in these situations is that if he is strong, he can lift you from the ground. If he accomplishes this, he can throw you to the ground and resume the assault, placing you in a much more difficult position to defend. You can also be

Grabbed While Standing

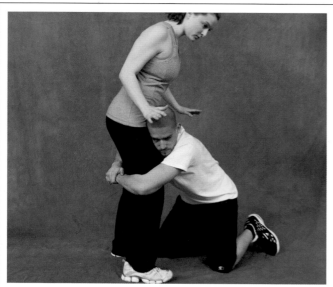

- Sometimes an attacker will grab around your legs when you are standing up.

- This can happen if you have disengaged from a wrestling match on the ground or if you are defending yourself on your feet, and he tries to tackle you.

- This is a dangerous situation because going to the ground will limit your options and put you at a disadvantage.

- Fight for your balance and do not allow him to hug your legs together.

Hips Forward, Legs Away

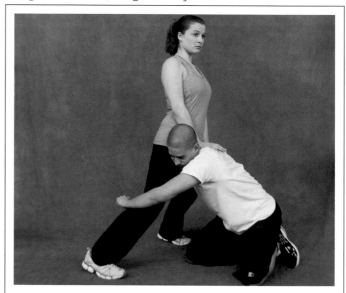

- As your attacker tries to bring your legs together, drive them apart to make it difficult for him to hug them both.

- Place your feet wide so that he cannot tip you off balance easily.

- Drive the hip forward and into him, making it harder to lift you or to get under your center of gravity. Use the strength of your back and glutes to fight back against him.

injured during your landing, especially if you strike your arms, spine, or head on the ground or nearby objects.

And if he is particularly strong, he may be able to lift you up and carry you from the scene. Abductions carry much higher risks than ordinary assault situations and should be treated as seriously as any lethal attack.

Fight to maintain your balance and stop him from establishing a position of strength under your hips. Drive him away and do not allow him to push, pull, or drag you to the ground.

ZOOM

Throughout this process you must remain balanced and heavy. Make yourself impossible to lift or topple by focusing your weight downward and driving your feet and knees wide. Catch your balance in your hands if necessary. Do not let him lift you up or topple you to the ground! It will not be so easy to escape a second time.

Push the Head Away

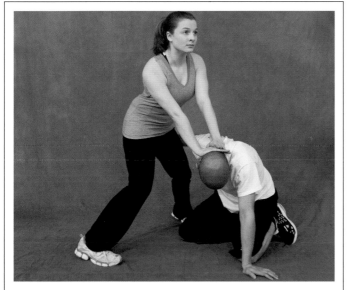

- Separate from him by pushing his head away. Extract your legs by pushing him away from them.

- Maintain your balance as you drive him off. Shove his head downward to make it difficult for him to follow you.

- You can use this as an opportunity to attack his eyes by getting your fingers into them as you push. You can also follow this by kicking or kneeing his head.

Danger of Being Lifted

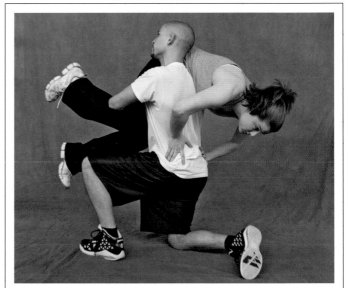

- If the attacker can bring your knees together, it will be much easier for him to take you down.

- With your balance compromised, he can tackle you to the ground or lift you up.

- This is a precarious situation because you have lost considerable control and are now exposed to much greater dangers.

- Keep your legs away from him at all costs. He should never be allowed to grab both legs at the same time.

STANDING & FIGHTING

No matter how the conflict begins, you must become aggressive as quickly as possible

This page shows a possible sequence of events beginning with a "victim" seated in front of a hostile aggressor.

Here our "victim," Hope, reacts immediately to her would-be assailant and delivers a kick to begin her defense. The kick doubles as both a distraction and a push to maintain distance between him and herself. Seeing him react to the

pain of the kick, she takes advantage of the short window of time to establish a neutral position: By standing up she has removed his advantage over her.

While she stands, Hope is evaluating her attacker to gauge his reaction to the kick and his intentions. In this case she judges that based upon his initial aggression and his current

KNACK SELF-DEFENSE FOR WOMEN

Kicking to Create Space

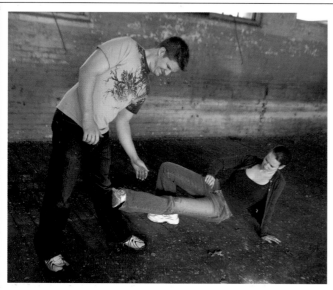

- Sitting in front of a standing attacker is not a desirable position.

- As her attacker becomes violent, Hope buys herself time to stand up and even the playing field before the situation becomes worse.

- Preparing to stand up in base, she places her weight on her hand and opposite foot and lifts herself from the ground.

- While protecting her personal space, she delivers a sharp kick to the knee to buy herself time.

Standing Up in Base

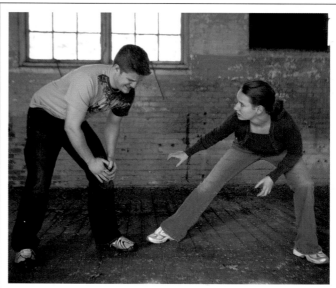

- When Hope sees that the kick bought her a moment to act, she brings her leg underneath her body and stands up in base.

- She can protect herself with her hands in the event that he tries to grab her as she stands up.

- As she stands, she watches her assailant the entire time and evaluates the situation.

- She needs to decide if she has the opportunity to leave or if he will continue the attack as he recovers.

body language, he will attempt to resume the assault as soon as he regains his composure. She takes advantage of his temporary distraction and brings the fight to him, taking hold of his upper body while his hands are down. Because he is not paying full attention to her, and because his hands are not protecting his head, it is easy for her to establish a strong grip on his neck.

She throws several strong knee strikes to his groin in this position, after which she will push him away and disengage fully.

ZOOM

When you reach your feet, you are at a critical point where you must evaluate the situation and decide what is appropriate. If you feel that you can safely exit the scene, take advantage of that option. If you feel that the danger persists and that your attacker will chase you and continue the assault, then you may need to take the upper hand in this moment of opportunity.

Entering the Clinch

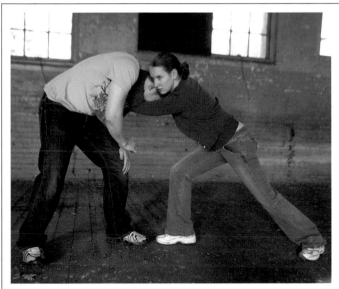

- Judging that he still intends her harm, Hope decides to take control of the situation by immediately grabbing onto his neck.

- Because he is still reacting to the pain in his knee, his head is down, and his neck is easily within reach.

- His moment of distraction provides an opportunity for Hope to enter the clinch range without much opposition.

- She establishes strong control over the neck to make it harder for him to recover and to defend against her strikes.

Knee to the Groin

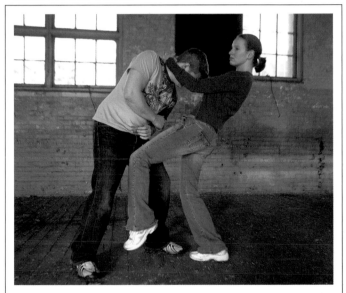

- Swinging her hips forward from their previous position, Hope drives a knee to the groin.

- She pulls down hard on his neck to bring him into the force of the blow. Doing this will increase her control over him and the force of the impact.

- She will throw several of these knees until she can see that he no longer intends to continue the assault, at which point she will push him away and run.

ESCAPING THE MOUNT

In a bad position, you must create as much space as possible

Being stuck underneath the mount is a desperate position. You must work quickly and aggressively to recover to a place where you can fight more effectively.

Here our "victim," Meagin, finds herself trapped underneath the mount. She selects a target that is within reach and will cause immense pain, and she bites her attacker on the nipple. She pulls and tears at him with her teeth as she hugs around the body so that it is difficult for him to pull away.

When he backs away to protect himself, this is the critical time for Meagin. If she misses this opportunity to extract herself from underneath him, she may find herself under an even more aggressive attacker in a few seconds.

Meagin scoots herself backward and frees her legs. She knows that the safety of the open guard position will allow her to defend space and keep him from pinning her again. By creating distance between his hips and her own, she can

Hug and Bite

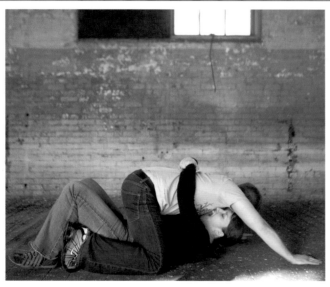

- In this sequence Meagin finds herself in a particularly difficult situation. No one wants to be trapped under the mount, and he may try to strike or choke her.

- Because of this fact, she wastes no time in taking the fight to her attacker. She establishes control over

his body by hugging her head close to his chest and biting the nipple.

- She bites hard and repeatedly to cause shock and intense pain. She knows he will be forced to give up his position if he wants to escape her bite.

Free Your Legs

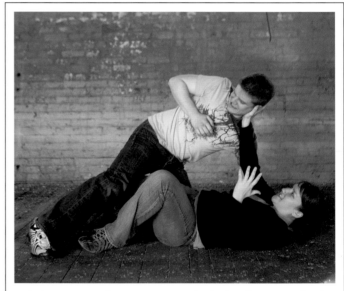

- As he reacts to the pain from her bite, she wastes no time in pushing him away with her hands and moving herself backward.

- She frees her left leg first and then her right, bringing both legs out from underneath him.

- In the brief moment that he spends reacting to the bite, she is able to turn the tables dramatically and bring strong pushing tools—her legs—in between the two of them.

bring her legs into play. The difference between the position of having her legs trapped under the mount and the position of being able to use her feet and knees freely after she has moved backward is tremendous.

With her legs free, she can play open guard until the opportunity presents itself to stand and engage or escape.

ZOOM

Escaping positions such as these takes a combination of timing, aggressiveness, and technical know-how. Students of Brazilian Jiu-Jitsu spend years perfecting the ability to move underneath difficult positions in order to escape. Although the sequence above is realistic and workable, anyone who wants to develop deeper ability in escaping is advised to seek out Brazilian Jiu-Jitsu training.

Feet on Hips

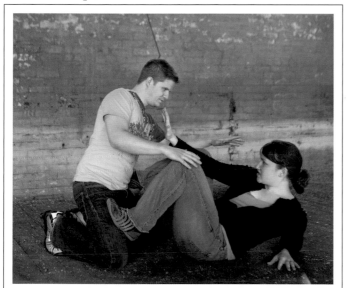

- By the time he realizes what has happened, Meagin has already established strong pushing motions in the open guard position and is working to stand up in base.

- Having started with almost no space between herself and her attacker, she has gained a tremendous amount of ground and placed several pushing tools in front of herself for protection.

- Doing this provides her the opportunity to get to her feet as he tries to recover.

Knee to the Head

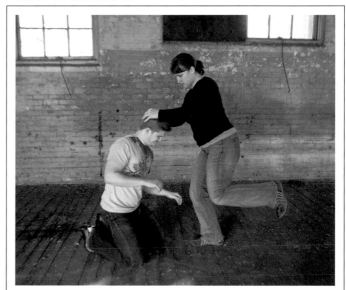

- Although Meagin reaches her feet before her attacker does, he continues to pursue her.

- She takes control of his head and aims a knee. By pulling him into its path, she can guarantee a solid strike.

- She is careful to avoid him as he tries to grab her legs and throws several quick knees to the head to take the fight out of him.

- As he finally stops trying to continue, she seizes the opportunity to run.

REENGAGING AFTER STANDING 1
Sometimes a grab is your opportunity to turn the tables in your favor

Here we see an example in which our "victim," Lena, has been grabbed while attempting to stand and escape from her attacker. Although this can be a dangerous situation, she turns it to her advantage by maintaining her balance.

When she feels him grab around her legs, Lena drives forward and establishes the top position. Although she wasn't able to break his grip, she managed to make the best of the situation by taking the opportunity to more effectively control him. By driving him off balance, she is able to take a dominant position and begin raining down punches and other strikes to finish the encounter.

The mount position is one where a fight can be quickly finished if the attacker simply will not relent. By striking in this position, Lena can put her full body weight into the downward punches and strikes, thanks to the assistance of gravity. By throwing many full-force punches, elbows, and

Grabbed by the Legs

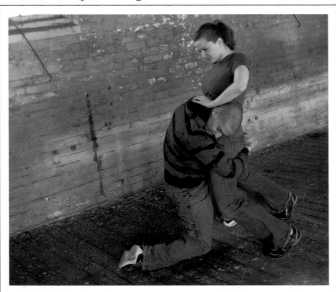

- As Lena stands up to escape, her attacker grabs her around the legs in order to pull her back down.

- Because he has caught her off guard, she is unable to drive her legs apart to stop him. This sometimes happens against a particularly fast or strong assailant.

- Now her balance is in jeopardy, and she must worry about being taken to the ground.

Driving to the Mount

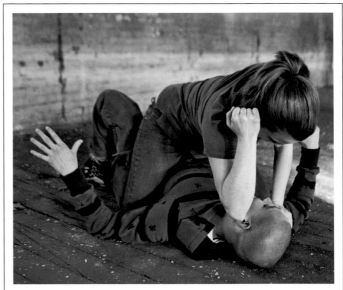

- Because she cannot stop the takedown from happening, Lena decides to capitalize on the situation and to take control as best she can.

- She drives forward into her attacker as he drags her down and steps over him into the mount position.

- Although he has succeeded in bringing her to the ground, she has managed to turn it into an opportunity to take control and try to end the encounter.

other strikes, she can overwhelm her attacker and knock him unconscious, injure him, or destroy his intent to continue fighting. In any of these cases, she should be able to put a stop to the danger here.

ZOOM

A similar sequence of events might take place if Lena has fully disengaged, but he is clearly still intent on pursuing her (or other bystanders). She might take it upon herself to reengage with him before he gets up to his feet, tackling him down into a position that affords her dominance and the ability to punish him with strikes, ending the situation safely for everyone else involved.

Punches from the Mount

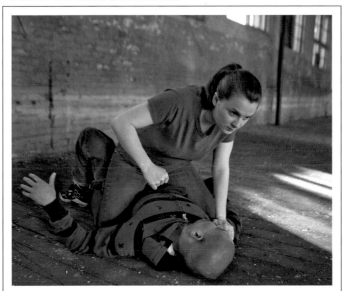

- Having established the mount position, Lena wastes no time. Her advantage may be brief, so she makes the most of it.

- As soon as she has her balance, Lena begins raining punches down at her attacker. Because she is on top, she can turn her hips into the punches, putting her weight behind them.

- Gravity also aids her as she punches downward, adding extra force to the impact.

- With his head against the ground, it is difficult for her attacker to avoid the strikes.

Elbows from the Mount

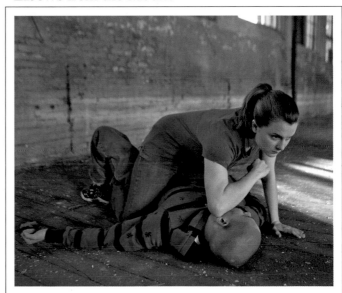

- Having met some success with her punches, Lena mixes in some elbow strikes.

- She knows that punching the sturdy bones of the skull can injure her hands, so as her attacker turns his head in an effort to avoid her punches, she switches to striking with her elbows.

- She continues throwing strikes in this position until it is clear that he no longer wishes to continue the assault.

REENGAGING AFTER STANDING 2

When you cannot mount from your takedown defense, you can often move to the side

In this example we see our "victim," Morgan, grabbed by an attacker as she attempts to create space and stand. By keeping her balance and driving him away, she is able to turn the tables and create a situation of advantage where she can end the encounter.

The key to Morgan's success here is that she drives him

off balance while retaining her own base. As she pushes his shoulders backward and to the side, he is unable to support himself. As he reaches the ground, she anchors to him and immediately begins striking his head before he can regroup and attempt to escape.

From the side it is more difficult to throw punches, although

KNACK SELF-DEFENSE FOR WOMEN

Grabbed around the Legs

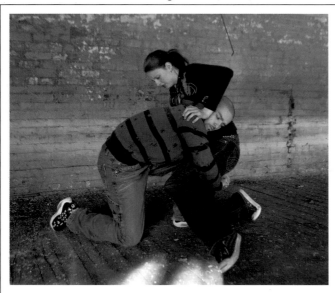

- As Morgan attempts to stand up and escape, her attacker grabs her legs to try to put her onto her back again.

- Because he has brought her almost all the way back to the ground, it will be difficult to step over and

mount, as in the previous sequence.

- Instead Morgan will catch her balance behind her on one foot and drive forward into her attacker.

Driving to the Side

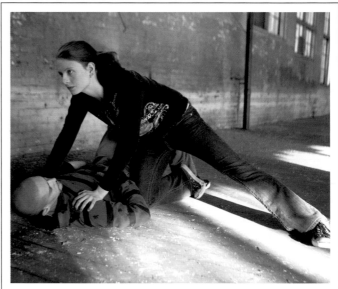

- As she pushes back into her assailant, Morgan is able to push his back to the ground.

- She places her knee beside his hip and controls his far shoulder so that it will be difficult for him to drive her off of him.

- Because she lacks the angle to step over and establish the mount, she instead moves to the side position, pinning him from there.

- Although she wanted to avoid coming back to the ground, she finds the opportunity to take control of the situation.

it can be done. Instead the weapons of choice are often elbows and knees. These allow you to keep your weight on your attacker and maintain your pulling motions, making it hard for him to escape while still allowing you to strike effectively.

Although the elbows will be used primarily to deliver short, choppy, stunning blows, the strikes to the head using the knee are real "fight-enders." Several knee strikes to the head will do tremendous damage and have the potential to finish the encounter.

Elbows to the Head

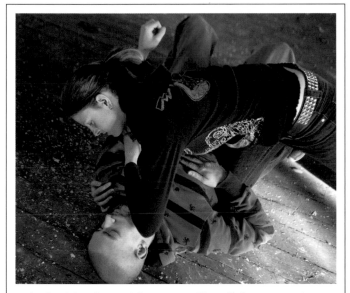

- As she drives her weight down onto him, Morgan begins to turn the tide by firing elbow strikes into his face.

- She hugs his shoulder so that he cannot push her away to avoid her strikes.

- She will throw several vicious strikes here to try to overwhelm him and to establish control.

- It will be hard for him to continue the assault while he is forced to defend himself.

Knees to the Head

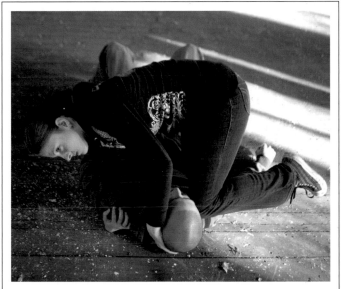

- As the situation turns to her favor, Morgan switches from elbow strikes to knee strikes.

- She grabs onto the far side of his head to pull him into the impact and to make sure that she connects accurately.

- Using the strong muscles of the hip, she throws strong, heavy knees to his head.

- Because of the danger of being pulled to the ground, Morgan wasted no time in ending this assault before it reached a point of no return.

PROTECTING SPACE

Keep your pushing tools in action when an attacker tries to push through your defenses

Here is an example of how the various tools to defend space are integrated in the face of an attacker who is determined to engage you.

Our "victim," Meagin, begins this sequence seated in the face of an aggressor who is initiating a violent situation. As he drives forward, she does a good job of establishing pushing motions early, even while he is still standing. Although she does this well, there are some cases in which a particularly aggressive or determined attacker will crash his way through your pushes in an attempt to take control.

Meagin continues with the pushing motions until he reaches close range, at which point she switches tactics

He Charges

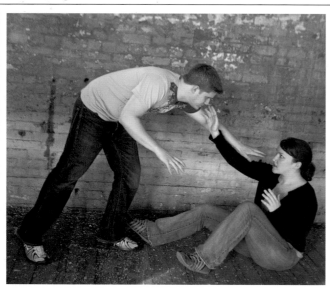

- In this example Meagin faces an attacker who is determined to reach her.

- He surprises her while she's sitting and comes running at her in an attempt to tackle her and pin her down.

- Meagin sees the situation develop and is ready to push him away with her hands and feet to protect the space between herself and him.

He Continues Driving Forward

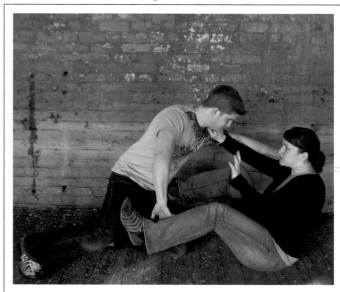

- Although Meagin pushes him back, her attacker fights tremendously to reach her.

- She continues scooting backward and pushing him away with every tool she can, but he continues gaining ground.

- He is persistent and aggressive and is strong enough to make his way closer and closer as she attempts to control the space.

suddenly, pulls him into the closed guard where she has more safety, and then proceeds to counterattack him viciously. The change from pushing to pulling followed by the change from simple pushing tools to painful attacking catches him off guard and allows her the time to reestablish pushing tools and get to her feet.

The ability to adapt that Meagin demonstrates is critical. She recognizes that her first attempts were not successful and immediately changes tack to another approach and a different set of skills.

He Closes the Distance

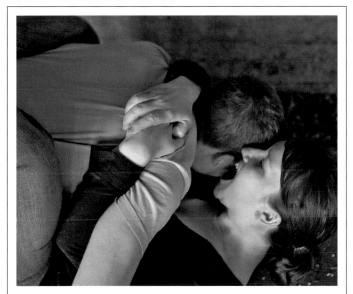

- As he fights his way past her defenses, Meagin realizes that she must change tactics to control the situation. She stops pushing him away and instead pulls him into the closed guard. She wraps her legs around his trunk and her arms around his upper body to control him.

- Having pulled him into a very close range, Meagin immediately starts viciously biting her attacker's face and neck.

- If he wants to be at such close distance, he will face the consequences of arriving there.

Reclaiming Space

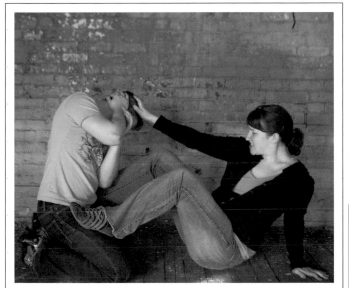

- As he reacts to the biting, Meagin senses an opportunity to reestablish her pushing tools.

- Because he is no longer driving forward, she places her feet on the hips and pushes him away. She has better success now that he

is trying to protect himself from her bite.

- If she has a sufficient window of time, she will stand up and make her escape or reengage from a better position away from the ground.

ESCAPING A RELENTLESS ATTACKER
How to disengage when he will not stop pursuing you

In some cases you may face an attacker who will not yield, no matter how many escape attempts you make. Even if you get to your feet and attempt to completely disengage, he will not relent.

In this example our "victim," Meagin, has fought off her attacker and gotten to her feet, but he will not stop trying to reengage and drag her back to the ground. She frees her leg by pushing on his head and then assesses her options. She

aims a kick at his head while making sure she does not offer him another opportunity to grab her leg. When she sees that the kick is successful but that he is still intent on pursuing her, she aims a stomp at the back of his head. As he collapses, no longer intent on continuing the fight, she takes the opportunity to run.

Meagin does a good job here of maintaining distance from her attacker. She wants to be sure that he cannot grab

He Will Not Stop

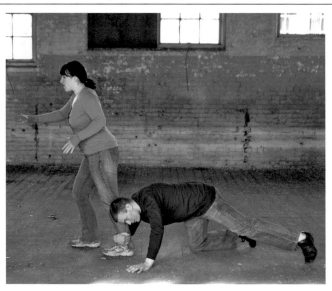

- In this example Meagin has already struck her assailant repeatedly and tried to make her escape but to no avail.

- Although she has struck him successfully, he is determined to continue, and as she attempts to

leave, he tries to renew the assault.

- In this situation, although it looks at first as though Meagin is the aggressor, she is defending herself from an attacker who refuses to stop.

Control the Head

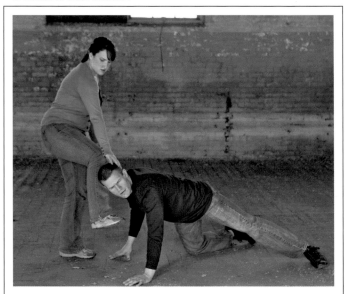

- As he grabs at her ankles, Meagin quickly pulls her foot away from his grasp.

- Seeing that he aims to pursue her, she places a hand on his head and pushes him down and away from her legs.

- She aims a soccer-style kick at his head while she pushes him away.

- She must be careful not to provide him an opportunity to grab her as she counters his attack.

her around the body or legs in an effort to drag her to the ground. By focusing on keeping his head away, she can provide herself some safety as she finishes the exchange.

Although this sequence may seem excessive out of context, remember that the key is to watch for signs that the attacker is no longer continuing the assault. Until that point it is necessary for you to do whatever you can to protect yourself because the attack is still under way. If that means kicking a man in the head while he's on the ground, so be it.

Stomp to the Head

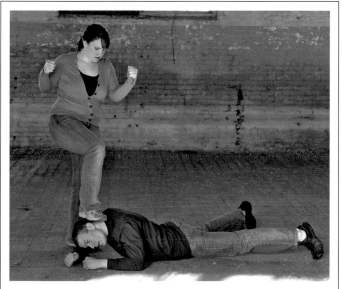

- Having met some success with her soccer kick, Meagin follows it up with a stomp to the back of the head.

- She continues this attack without allowing him to return to the assault.

- She must take advantage of the opportunity afforded to her by the successful kick.

- One or more quick stomps to the hands, head, or neck should dissuade him from continuing.

Escape Finally

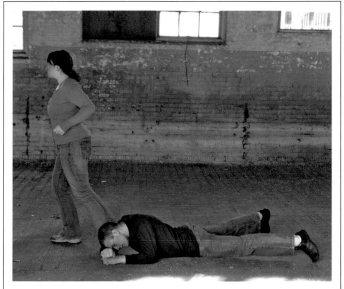

- After a few stomps, she sees that finally his desire to fight has gone.

- As soon as she judges that he will not pursue her, she immediately turns to run.

- There is no need to continue her response if the danger has ended for herself and others in the immediate area. She will now seek the help of security or law enforcement and consult medical help if she is injured.

LETHAL INTENT VS NEGOTIATION
Why do attackers use weapons, and what does it mean when they do?

Situations involving weapons fall into two main categories: lethal intent and negotiation. In the first category, someone out there in the world is targeting you personally. This person intends to find you and kill you. These are rare situations, and the primary recommendation is that you not make enemies in the first place.

Most situations, however, fall into the second category. These are situations in which the assailant uses a weapon as leverage in a negotiation: He intends to take advantage of you in some way, and the weapon serves as the reason why you should give him what he wants.

It doesn't much matter what the negotiation involves.

Confronted with a Weapon

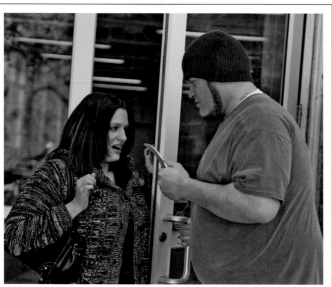

- Weapons are often used as a way of asserting control in order to take advantage of you in some way.

- Because the weapon acts as a "trump card," it forces you to comply with whatever the demands are.

- This is a dangerous situation and not to be taken lightly. You must assume that someone with a weapon is willing to use it.

Do Not Escalate

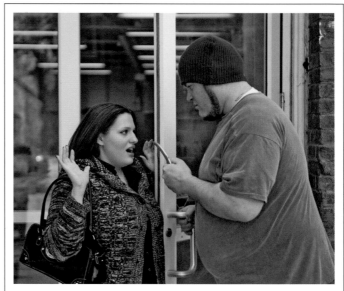

- Try to remain as calm as possible, even though it will be difficult.

- Moderate your speech and body language to avoid escalating the conflict and increasing the risk to yourself and others.

- It's important that you recognize how high the threat level is here: It's dangerous to be overconfident, especially if you have had some training.

- Physical intervention should be an absolute last resort. Mistakes can have tremendous consequences.

"Give me your wallet." "Hand over your car keys." "Take off your clothes." "Open the vault." All of these are situations in which he intends to force your cooperation by brandishing a weapon.

The first good news is that if he merely intended to attack you with the weapon, he probably would have done so already. It makes little sense to demand a wallet and *then* shoot someone because if he shoots you first he could just take the wallet without the trouble of asking you. Provided you do not escalate the situation or give him reason to attack you, it should be possible to survive the situation.

The second good news is that he is looking for your cooperation. There is some action expected on your part, and in that lies the kernel of opportunity for you to act.

In most situations it is unwise to start a fight with someone armed. Better courses of action involve complying with the demand but distancing yourself from the weapon. Some situations may also offer the chance to escape before they play out more violently.

Comply within Reason

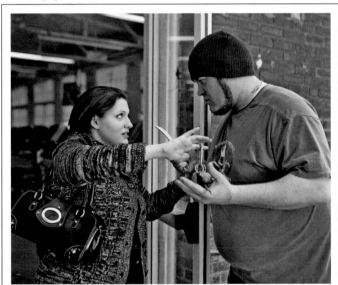

- Although you may not like the idea of cooperating, it is often your safest option.

- Judge the situation carefully. If you think your attacker will leave you unharmed if you give him what he wants, it's worth trying.

- If this person is really after only your wallet, car keys, or other belongings, hand them over.

- Do you really own anything as irreplaceable as your own life?

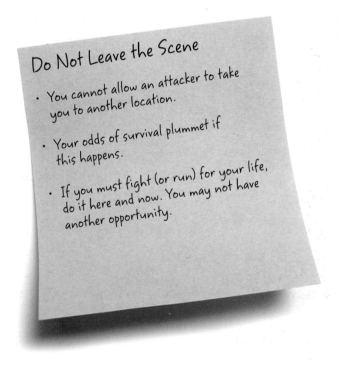

Do Not Leave the Scene

- You cannot allow an attacker to take you to another location.

- Your odds of survival plummet if this happens.

- If you must fight (or run) for your life, do it here and now. You may not have another opportunity.

169

CARJACKING
Comply with an armed attacker while separating yourself from danger

Our policy with most armed attackers will be "comply but create distance." We will walk a delicate tightrope of cooperating with the demands while developing safe distance between ourselves and the weapon.

In this case our "victim," Meg, is exiting her car as she is approached by an armed assailant. He demands that she exit

the vehicle and hand over her keys. She understands that the biggest priority will be to create safe distance between herself and the knife. She will need to keep from agitating him while she is so close to the threat and to create an opportunity to move herself away from both the weapon and her vehicle.

By keeping calm and offering to give him the keys, she

Approached in Your Vehicle

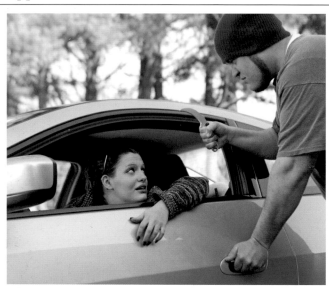

- In this example we'll show one method of handling a situation with an armed attacker.

- Here Meg is about to exit her car when she is ordered out by an assailant with a knife.

- In some cases she might be able to drive away to escape her attacker.

- Here he has come so close that she lacks the time to start the car and get away. She will need to proceed carefully.

Keep Things Calm

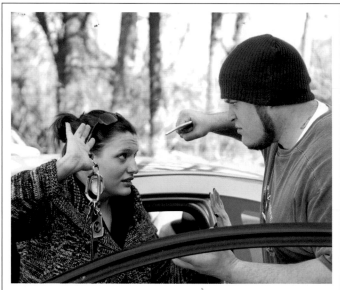

- Meg does her best not to escalate the situation. She cooperates with the demand to exit her vehicle, but she monitors the situation for an opportunity to escape.

- The most difficult thing about this situation is the close physical proximity.

- She will not be able to avoid coming into close contact with her attacker.

creates the opportunity to separate herself from what he's demanding. She can put him in a position to choose between threatening her and taking the car, reassuring him that he's getting what he wanted.

"Comply but create distance" is an important policy because it makes the situation win-win. He takes what he's after and allows her to escape. Although some situations will not play out in this way, the same concepts should be our guide. Offer to cooperate with the demand while creating safety for yourself.

ZOOM

Beyond the obvious reason that her life is more valuable than her car, Meg moves away from her vehicle for a second reason: The situation will be much more dire if she hands over her keys and then is forced back into the vehicle with him. Leaving with him escalates her risk significantly. She moves far away from the car so that he cannot force her back in easily.

Creating Separation

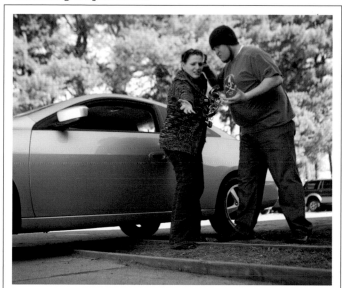

- Meg makes it clear that she is cooperating with the demand.

- She speaks clearly and calmly as she tosses the keys to the ground. She must not give the impression of antagonizing him or being uncooperative.

- Here she has found a way to comply with the demand for her keys without keeping herself at risk.

- This forces her assailant to choose between keeping her close and fetching the keys.

Opportunity to Escape

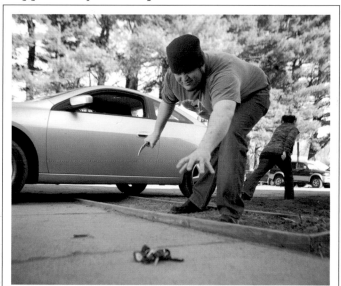

- As she watches him go to grab the keys, Meg wastes no time in running. She does not need to wait around for the situation to become worse.

- She has done a good job of keeping the situation calm and of creating distance between herself and the armed attacker.

- Within the attacker's demand, she found the kernel of opportunity that allowed her to escape. She found a way to give him what he wanted and to achieve her goal—safe escape—too.

BLUNT & FLEXIBLE WEAPONS

Tools used for impact or entanglement operate primarily within a certain distance

Blunt weapons are primarily instruments of impact, whereas flexible weapons are a mix of entanglement and trauma tools. Both of these can be dangerous elements in play during an assault.

Blunt weapons (also called "impact weapons") include anything, from a carefully designed weapon to a random object picked up off the ground that can be used to strike someone. Some blunt weapons (such as brass knuckles) create a more forceful impact, whereas others (such as a stick) allow the strike to reach a farther distance. Many items in this group fulfill some mix of the two elements—for example, a baseball bat.

Many impromptu weapons will fall into this group. You can

Impact and Flexible Weapons

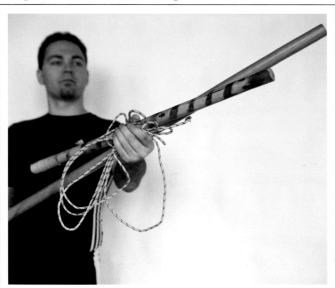

- Impact weapons include a broad variety of objects: sticks, bats, canes, batons, bricks, brass knuckles, and many more.

- Virtually any solid object can become a blunt weapon if wielded by a motivated individual.

- Flexible weapons include ropes, chains, whips, and the like. Although some of them are used to entangle you, others (such as a rope with a weight on the end) may also be impact weapons.

Inside the Arc

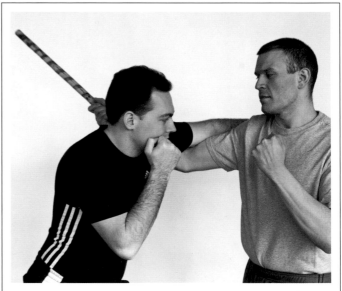

- Blunt weapons are used because of their impact abilities. Their length also extends the assailant's reach.

- It's important to be in one of two places against a blunt weapon: too far away or too close.

- Standing in the arc of the swing is the worst place to be because the weapon is at its most dangerous there.

- When the time is right, move inside the arc so that the weapon will pass behind you.

pick up a chair, a piece of wood, a hammer, and so on. Each of these can be a valuable striking tool to use during an assault because it increases the range of your strikes, the force of your strikes, or both.

Flexible weapons are more commonly used to entangle, although they can also be impact tools. Some flexible weapons are weighted at one end, allowing them to develop momentum if swung at someone. These include weighted chains or ropes with an object on the end or even the clichéd sock with a bar of soap inside.

Other flexible weapons, including ropes, chains, duct tape, fishing line, electrical wire, and zip ties, are used to entangle or bind. These weapons have a primary danger of limiting your movement so that you cannot escape further assault but have secondary dangers as well. Thin materials, such as fishing line and so on, can create permanent nerve damage if used to bind the skin, for instance, in the tying of arms and legs. They can also be used as choking devices if applied around the neck, which is a third major danger when dealing with flexible weapons.

Hugging the Arms

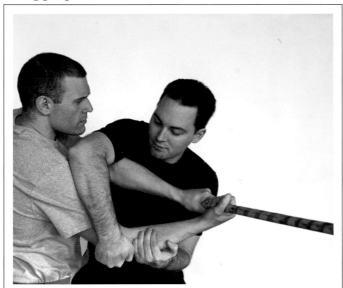

- Although the danger is not as severe, you are still at risk in close quarters against a blunt weapon.

- When possible, tie up the attacker's arms to make it difficult to use the weapon. Hugging the back of the arm will make striking you difficult.

- After you are in this position, waste no time launching a counterattack of knees, headbutts, elbows, and whatever else is available to you.

- The best way to disarm a weapon is to cause significant trauma to the person holding it.

Entangled by Flexible Weapons

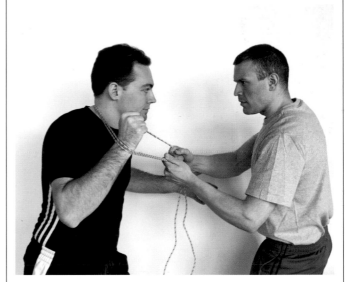

- The primary dangers of flexible weapons are the risk of becoming entangled.

- These dangers are particularly severe if the weapon is around your neck because you can become the victim of a choke.

- Flexible weapons can also be used to bind you temporarily while the assault takes place or for longer periods of time in order to abduct you from the scene or leave you incapacitated.

EDGED WEAPONS

How to address blades of all shapes and sizes

Blades are widely available tools that often come to mind readily when discussing armed assault. Blades are among the most dangerous weapons you can encounter when protecting yourself.

First and foremost, blades are lethal tools. A thrust or stab to the body or major bloodway of the arms and legs can be fatal. You must take the utmost precaution when encountering a blade of any shape or size.

Sharp or edged weapons take many forms, including many objects that were not intended as weapons. Anything sharp enough to pierce the skin, including broken glass, razor blades, a sturdy pen, a pair of scissors, nails, drill bits, and so on, can be used in an attack.

One of the things that makes blades so dangerous is that they can be used repeatedly. They do not run out of ammunition. They are always dangerous.

Single or Double Edged

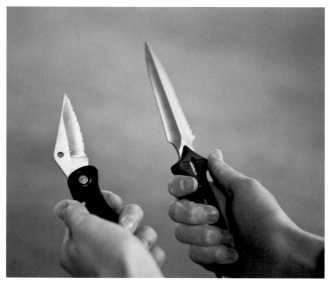

- The two main types of knives are single edged and double edged. With a single-edged knife, you can find safety along the back side of the blade. Against double-edged knives, the only safe sides are the flat ones.

- Blades can vary in length

from a few inches, such as a razor blade, to multiple feet, such as a machete.

- In addition to knives, edged weapons include swords, nails, spikes, razor blades, box cutters, broken glass, and anything else sharp enough to cut, pierce, or puncture.

Stay Out of Range

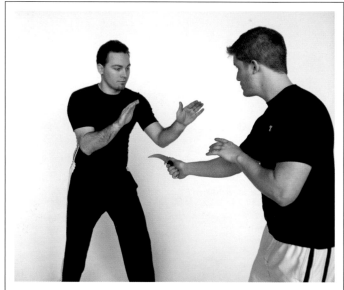

- The primary strategy against a blade or other cutting tool should be to keep yourself far enough away that it cannot reach you.

- Engaging a blade is difficult because it can do tremendous damage and does not need to be reloaded.

- Unfortunately many attackers will often conceal the weapon until they are close to you or have already attacked you with it.

- You may not even realize that an edged weapon was involved until after the assault is over.

It is extremely dangerous to try to take a blade away from somebody. Most blades allow the wielder to grip the handle firmly, leaving us with no safe area to grab—only the blade itself. When you must make contact with it, do so at the back edge (if it has one) or the flat side. But even then, this provides only temporary safety.

Your primary strategies must be to avoid the weapon entirely, to control the attacker's wrist if you cannot avoid him, and to fight with a weapon of your own whenever possible. You must take any advantage that you can in this situation and cause as much injury and trauma as possible while avoiding the blade. Traditional disarm techniques are an option only for fanatics who practice them daily. Your plan should be to avoid, and, failing that, it should be to aggressively control and attack the knife wielder.

Contact the Flat Side

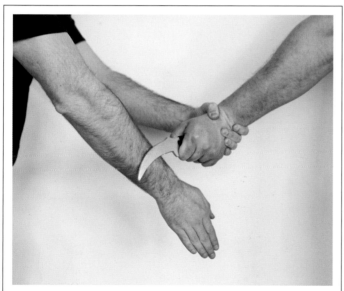

- If you must make contact with the weapon, the safest place is along the flat side.

- Some martial arts, especially many from the Philippines, specialize in the offense and defense of edged weapons.

- It takes many years of intense training to develop the skills to successfully survive an encounter against a knife-wielding attacker. Do not approach the situation lightly!

Controlling the Weapon

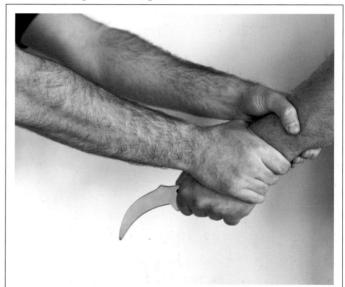

- Your priority is to secure the weapon arm and not let go. Hold it as though your life depends on it—because it just might.

- While holding the arm, use any other tools that you can, including headbutts, knee strikes, foot stomps, and shin kicks. Do as much damage as possible in order to loosen his grip on the knife.

- If he drops the blade, do not stop to pick it up. Instead move him away from it.

FIREARMS

Guns pose a significant threat and are not to be taken lightly

Firearms are the most common representative of modern projectile weapons, which include thrown weapons ranging from rocks to ninja stars, launching systems including bows and arrows, crossbows, and firearms, and aerosolized weapons such as pepper spray and Mace. Although all of these are dangerous tools, none of them commands the authority in today's world that is held by firearms.

Defensive actions are difficult in the face of a firearm because of the high levels of danger and stress involved. Although fantasies of disarming a person with a firearm may seem glamorous, the reality of facing a gun is a terrible situation. Do whatever you can to avoid the situation entirely.

Types of Firearms

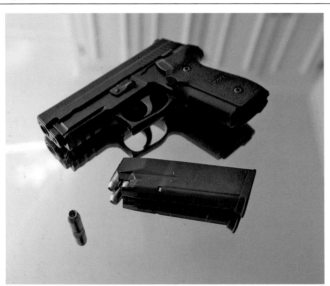

- For self-defense purposes, pistols are our primary concern because their ability to be concealed makes them ubiquitous.

- Pistols are divided into two types: revolvers (which have a rotating cylinder that houses the bullets) and semi-automatics (which automatically load the next bullet after firing).

- Modern long guns include rifles (which shoot one bullet at a time) and shotguns (which expel many types of ammunition, including packets of shot).

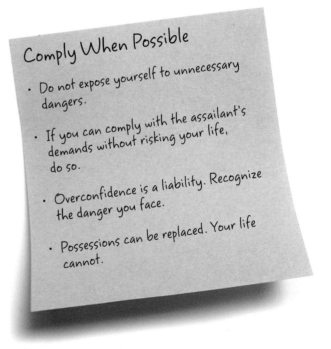

Comply When Possible

- Do not expose yourself to unnecessary dangers.

- If you can comply with the assailant's demands without risking your life, do so.

- Overconfidence is a liability. Recognize the danger you face.

- Possessions can be replaced. Your life cannot.

If you are considering owning a firearm for personal or home protection, be sure to train appropriately. Learn to handle it, to accurately fire it, and to fix it when it jams. If you are going to draw your weapon, you must be willing and able to shoot the weapon. Also, store and lock your weapon appropriately to avoid accidents. This is particularly important if you have children in the home.

Defensive action against a firearm should be taken only as a last resort. The danger is real and severe. There is no room for mistakes, and there can be consequences for you and for others nearby. Disarming weapons is a task reserved for fanatics who train daily under stressful conditions. It is not to be attempted in anything less than the worst of situations.

Deciding to Act

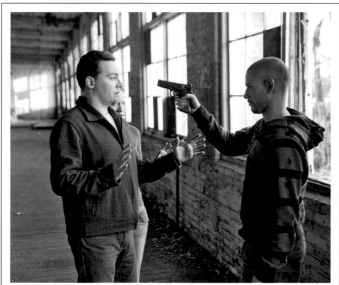

- The decision to act when confronted by a firearm is not one to be taken lightly.

- Even people with many years of training for such encounters should not engage an armed assailant unless absolutely necessary.

- If you sense, in the situation, that no matter what you do, your attacker intends to shoot you, then it's time to act. You must work quickly and decisively. There is little room for error.

The Line of Fire

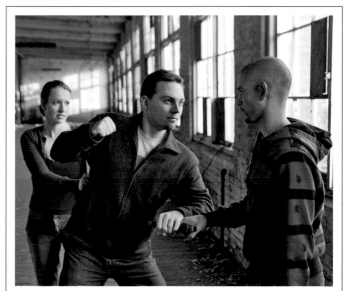

- If you decide to confront an armed attacker, work to redirect the weapon so that you (and any bystanders) are clear of the line of fire.

- Redirect the gun barrel off of your body in the shortest line available. Be sure to avoid turning it onto your companions or others.

- You do not have to be faster than a bullet, only faster than a trigger finger.

- Control the weapon and immediately attack the assailant. The danger must be controlled and neutralized.

ANTIDEPLOYMENT METHODS
Early action is always the better choice—when you have one

By recognizing the threat of a weapon in the preliminary stages, you can act before the threat fully develops. Learn to watch for movements that indicate deployment of a weapon—they are typically done with the attacker's dominant hand.

These actions can include reaching into a back pocket, into a boot or pants leg, or inside the breast of a jacket. When you see these actions, understand that they may indicate the presence of a weapon and your attacker's intent to use it.

The actions you should take when you see imminent deployment are the same simple, highly effective tools that you always use. However, the tricky part is training yourself to recognize the appropriate moment the instant it occurs.

If you can prevent the assailant from reaching his pocket or from withdrawing the weapon, you can limit the threat level of the encounter. This can be accomplished by attacking

Recognizing Deployment

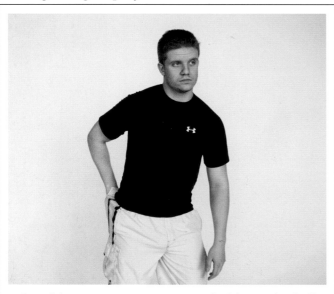

- One of the most important actions to watch for in an assault is the first sign that a weapon will be involved.

- When an attacker reaches behind his back, this is a sign that he will produce something. Typically you can assume that it will be a weapon.

- You don't know what he'll withdraw, but you can be fairly sure you don't want to know.

- When you see this motion—the hand going into the pocket—it's time to intercede immediately.

Eye Poke during Deployment

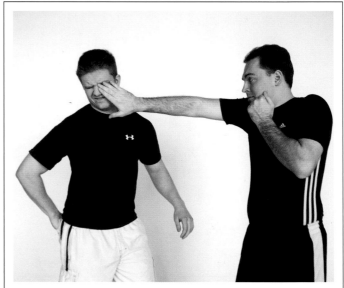

- If you see the hand disappear, one of the first things you should attack is the eye.

- Causing pain may buy you the time to distance yourself from him before the weapon is produced.

- Causing pain may even interrupt him as he tries to retrieve the weapon.

- Train yourself to recognize the action of deployment and to respond immediately. The time here is measured in fractions of a second.

vulnerable targets or by entangling his arm so that he cannot deploy his weapon.

If you find yourself engaged with someone at close range who attempts to deploy a weapon, cause as much trauma as possible while tying up the arms. You must work quickly to end this fight, or else you may yet wind up on the wrong end of a weapon.

ZOOM

When you see the movements that indicate weapon deployment, you will not yet know what kind of weapon he has. It doesn't make a difference. Whatever comes out of that pocket will not be good for you. Do you really want to wait and find out what it is? Spring into action the instant you see his hand approach his pocket.

Groin Kick during Deployment

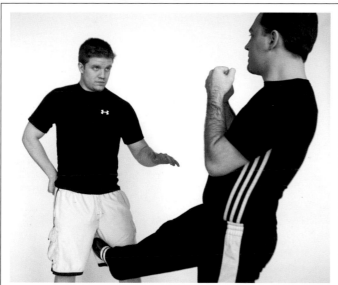

- If the range is slightly farther, it will be difficult to land the eye jab in time to stop him from deploying his weapon.

- Instead use a kick to the groin. Kicking will grant you a longer reach, eliminating the need to get closer to him.

- If he does successfully deploy his weapon, you will be glad to have had the extra distance between yourself and him.

- If you cannot keep him from arming himself, keep him at a distance.

Stopping the Deployment

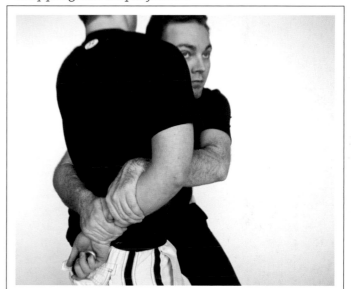

- If you are close enough, you can stop him from withdrawing his weapon by entering the clinch range.

- Bring your ear to his chest and wrap both arms around him. Grab his forearm tightly with both hands.

- If his hand hasn't reached his pocket yet, you can keep it from reaching. If he already has a hold of his weapon, you can use this wrap to stop him from deploying it.

- In this position strike and do as much damage as possible. Beware of his free hand.

179

DEALING WITH WEAPONS

PROTECTING OTHERS

When other lives are on the line, quick and decisive action is absolutely necessary

Protecting other people can be difficult. You cannot manage those persons' decisions or behavior, so you must control the situation as best you can to keep harm away from them.

If you can deescalate the situation, this is always for the best. But if you cannot, you will need to create a barrier between your companions and the attacker. Take the initiative in order to guide the situation before it develops momentum in the wrong direction. Steer the conflict away from your companions and when possible create a clear path for them to exit safely.

Protecting Your Companions

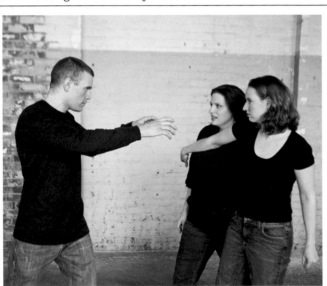

- When protecting others, you must move into action as quickly as possible.

- Assess the threat. Is there only one attacker or more? Where are you most needed? What is the biggest risk to you and to your companions?

- Although it is noble to stand up for others, do not put yourself at unnecessary risk. Who will protect them if you are injured and cannot continue to fight?

Create a Barrier

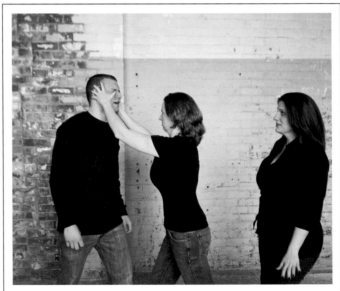

- Take control of the situation immediately. You cannot afford to underestimate the risk.

- Here we see our "victim," Hope, drive forward and grab her attacker's head in order to control him. She cannot wait for him to determine the course of action. Instead she dictates the action.

- By taking control of him, you maneuver the danger away from others. Passivity on your part offers him the opportunity to attack someone else. Seize the advantage and do not give it up!

Clear an Escape Path

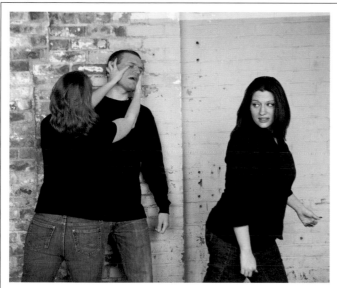

- The first priority when defending others should be to clear a path for their safe escape.

- When your attacker is between your companions and the exit, try to move him from their path to create an opportunity for them to get away.

- You may not be able to keep the exit clear for long, so be sure to communicate with your friends as you act.

- Give short, clear instructions. "Run *now*!"

When Escape Is Impossible

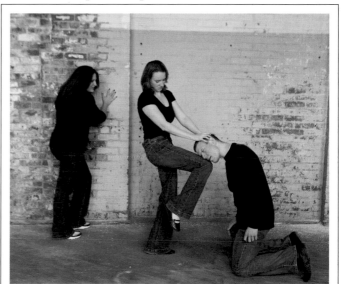

- In some situations there may not be a way to clear a path of safe escape for your companions.

- In these situations you must take the fight out of your attacker. He must be unwilling (or unable) to continue the assault. You must injure him, knock him uncon-

scious, or otherwise stop him from continuing.

- You must be extremely aggressive in these situations. When you protect yourself and others, everyone's safety is at stake. Use the most effective tools at your disposal, even if they are severe.

MULTIPLE ASSAILANTS
More than one attacker makes a tough situation even tougher

A common question at self-defense workshops is, "How should I handle a situation with multiple attackers?"

The short answer is this: Learn to handle one attacker before you can learn to take on several.

That isn't the whole story, of course. But it does raise an important point that shouldn't be overlooked: Fighting two attackers is more than twice as difficult as fighting one attacker. And one attacker is plenty difficult.

With multiple assailants you must avoid situations in which they can gang up on you and fight you together. Footwork and movement will be the most critical components in your defense, so that you can stay out of the middle of the group. Resist the tendency to overcommit to one attacker by clinching or grappling with him. Avoid going to the ground at all costs. The last place you want to be is stuck on the ground while several people attack you at once.

Keeping Everyone in Sight

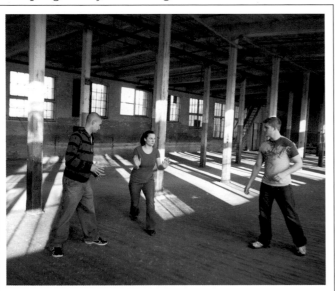

- The first priority when facing multiple attackers is to keep everyone in view.

- Do not allow yourself to be placed into a position in which you cannot see one or more assailants.

- If you lose visual contact, it will become almost impos-

sible to respond appropriately to attacks. The key to good defense is awareness.

- Move into a position where everyone is in view. Use your peripheral vision to watch everyone rather than looking back and forth from one to the other.

Move to the Outside

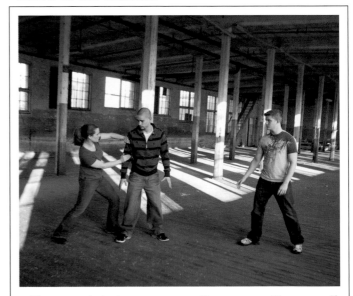

- The next priority is to move so that you are not between your attackers.

- Circle around to the outside and flank one of them. Doing this forces them to engage you one at a time instead of simultaneously.

- If you can, position yourself so that they appear to be in a line in front of you. This means one will be in the other's way.

- Use the environment to your advantage. Make it hard for them to coordinate their efforts.

When fighting against multiple attackers, you must take every single advantage available to you. Fight with a weapon. Be vicious. Take the initiative. Use your environment to its fullest. Exit at the first opportunity.

ZOOM

How did you wind up in this situation? What decisions did you make (or fail to make) that ended with your being surrounded by multiple attackers? We don't ask these questions as a way of casting blame, but we ask them rhetorically to remind ourselves that events are part of a timeline and that we have the ability to influence how events unfold.

Avoid the Middle

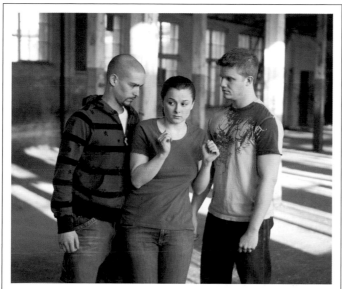

- If you get stuck in the center, you run the risk of being blindsided and overwhelmed.

- There is too much to deal with in the middle because attackers can gang up on you while you try to deal with them.

- Likewise, avoid being dragged to the ground at all costs. Positions that overly commit you into one place will be extremely hazardous against more than one assailant.

- Keep moving!

Find an Advantage

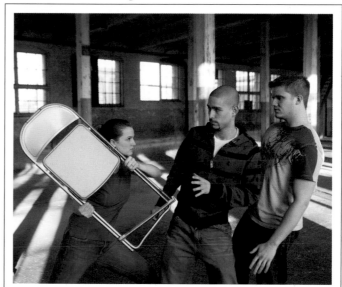

- Because you're fighting with a significant deficit, you should find and use anything you can to even the odds.

- If you carry a weapon, it's time to deploy it. If you don't, you need to find one.

- Throw dirt or a drink into someone's eyes. Push one of them into the other's path.

- Find something to give you an advantage—any advantage.

UNSAFE ENVIRONMENT

Sometimes your surroundings can limit your opportunity to defend yourself

The factor that defines your readiness in a crisis is your level of awareness. In the beginning we focus on your awareness of your own self—of your own strengths, weaknesses, and limitations. Through training we build your awareness until you no longer need to consciously examine yourself—you do this automatically.

Next we focus on training you to be aware of another person—your attacker. You will learn to be aware of his movements, his body language, his intentions. You will see what he is doing and how he is doing it. You will start to accurately predict these things based on early indications before they fully develop.

On Unsteady Terrain

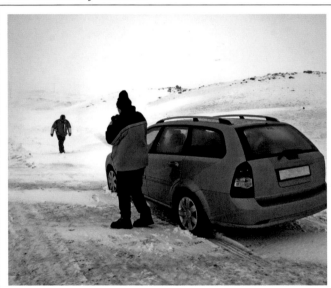

- Some environments, such as mud, ice, sand, and uneven ground, present difficulties in establishing your balance.

- If you can't keep your footing, it's nearly impossible to hit someone hard. You need the ability to push your weight off the ground in order to generate power in your strikes.

- Similarly, it is difficult to prevent someone from taking you to the ground if you cannot keep your balance.

- If you can't keep your footing, you also can't escape safely.

In the Stairway

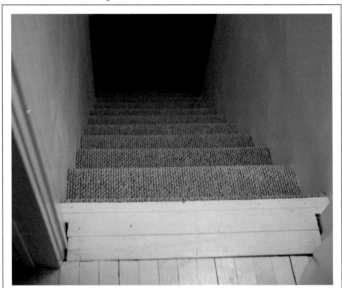

- Stairs are an example of an environmental hazard that you must consider while defending yourself.

- Fighting off an attacker too close to the top of a staircase can have dangerous consequences if you fall.

- Likewise, defending yourself in the middle of the staircase can be difficult because it places you slightly above or below your attacker and often with limited room to move or directions to run.

- Be aware of the hazards and limitations that your environment offers.

The next stage is to be aware of yourself and your attacker simultaneously. You must see how the interactions unfold, how he reacts to you, and how you react to him.

After you can do this successfully, you will expand your awareness to include your environment. Become aware of its dangers and its assets. See the things that harm you and help you or that harm and help your attacker.

Lastly, become simultaneously aware of yourself, your attacker, and your environment. See the situation in its totality and see how the pieces interact. Predict the play between these agents and any other agents as well. Be aware of what surrounds you.

Different environments will provide a variety of risks to you in a crisis. Some factors, such as fires and electrical currents, are obvious, whereas others, such as stairs, narrow passageways, confined spaces, and dead ends, may not be.

Items in your environment may be obstacles to one person and tools to another. Where one person sees a wall, another might see a window within reach. Learn to engage your environment and use its features to your advantage.

Too Close to Traffic

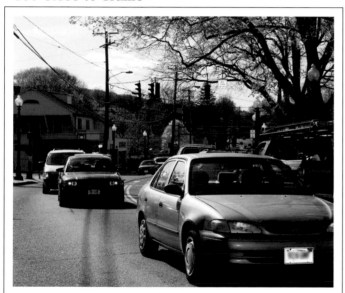

- Defending yourself in a roadway puts you at risk of being struck by a car.

- Are you too close to the street? Are you in danger of being struck by passing traffic? This is an example of a severe hazard that can change by the second.

- Other environments with similar intermittent risks include train or subway tracks and some types of electrical, heat, gas, and water passageways.

In Confined Spaces

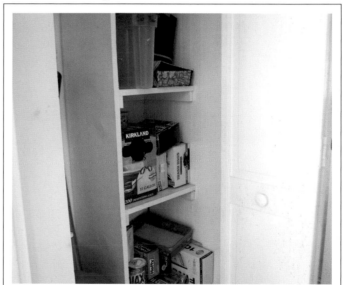

- Small, confined spaces present risks because movement in them can be difficult, whether you are fighting or escaping.

- In small spaces such as these, you cannot avoid many attacks. You will be forced to confront your attacker head on.

- Even if you are not claustrophobic, you may experience additional panic if you are forced to fight in a small, enclosed space.

FINDING A WEAPON
In a crisis almost anything can be used to give you an advantage

It's important to equalize the odds in any violent encounter. You don't know who this person is or what he knows. You don't know what he's armed with or how many people are involved. Assume the worst. Find a weapon that you can use and find it quickly.

If you don't carry a weapon of any kind, you'll need to find something in your environment that is useful to you. It can be something on your person or something you grab. Anything

can be useful if you approach it properly. Are you carrying a pen or pencil? How about your keys? Could you throw your cell phone into someone's face or hit him with your purse?

Do you have anything in your pockets that can be thrown into his face, such as loose change, receipts, business cards, or the like? Could you grab a fistful of dirt, rocks, grass, gravel, or anything in your environment that you can use?

Are you wearing anything that you can remove quickly,

Pens and Pencils

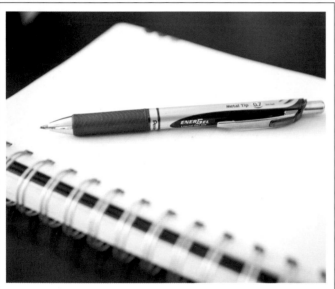

- Most people carry a pen or pencil in their pocket or bag.

- A pen or pencil can be used as a sharp instrument with which you can stab your attacker.

- Although this may seem extreme in some cases, fac-

ing an armed or otherwise dangerous assailant calls for you to use anything at your disposal.

- You can also ball up your fist around a pen and use it as a blunt striking tool by hitting with the top or bottom of your fist.

Your Keys

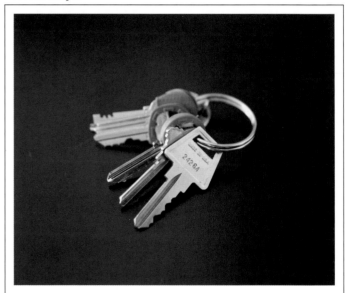

- It has long been conventional wisdom that your keys are a great weapon for self-defense.

- Strangely, it is often recommended that you make a fist around your keys, with a key sticking out between each finger. It is difficult, however, to imagine having

the time to do this during an assault.

- Instead grab your keys in your fist and strike with them all. Or hold one key between your thumb and forefinger and use it as a striking or cutting tool.

such as a belt, a hat, or a jacket? Are there drinks in your hand or nearby, such as a bottle of water or sports drink? What about hot beverages such as a cup of coffee or alcoholic drinks? These will have a more severe effect.

Use the environment to your advantage. Can you stand behind a door and slam it into him as he approaches? Can you pick up a chair or a book or anything else?

What is nearby? Are there items that you would find in a kitchen, such as knives? Are there tools around, such as hammers, screwdrivers, or drill bits?

In the end you can use anything in your environment, even if it's the last thing you might think to grab. Create a way to use it.

Hot Cup of Coffee

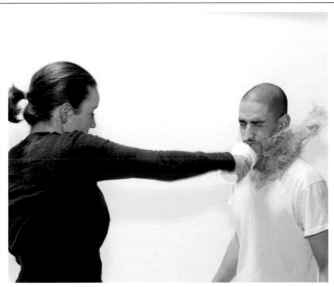

- Sometimes the best impromptu weapons are the ones that few people might think about.

- Many things can be used to startle, surprise, and distract an attacker if thrown into his face. Water, drinks, dirt, coins, and anything else that will scatter in the air are particularly valuable in this way.

- Some things (such as coffee or dirt) can also irritate the eyes, adding potency if you toss or spit them into someone's face.

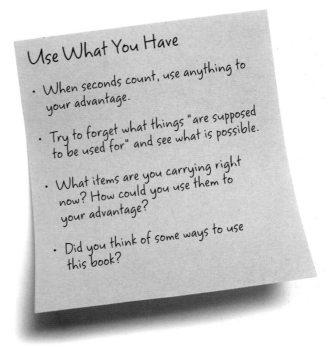

Use What You Have

- When seconds count, use anything to your advantage.

- Try to forget what things "are supposed to be used for" and see what is possible.

- What items are you carrying right now? How could you use them to your advantage?

- Did you think of some ways to use this book?

INSIDE A MOVING CAR
When trapped in a confined area, keep as much distance as you can

Escaping an assault in a moving vehicle is a challenge. You must make careful choices to take the path of greatest safety.

Certainly your priority is to escape the vehicle when you can. Depending on the severity of the situation, you might choose to bail out when it's still moving. Curl yourself into a ball and try to roll with the impact if the car is moving.

In lower-risk situations, you might wait until the vehicle stops before you make a quick exit. Be prepared to open the door and escape at the first opportunity. You may not have much time.

One important decision to make is whether you should wear your seatbelt. Wearing it means it will take more time for you to exit the vehicle, but not wearing it puts you at greater risk if the vehicle stops suddenly. If you are in the passenger seat and defending yourself against the driver, you

Legs between the Two of You

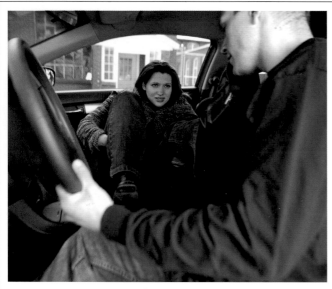

- Maintain distance between yourself and your assailant by placing your feet and knees between the two of you.

- This position can be used defensively to keep him away or offensively to kick at him.

- Brace your back against the door, provided it's closed securely.

- If you're in the back seat and protecting yourself from someone in the front seat, place yourself directly behind him and brace yourself against the back of your seat.

Hold the Door Handle

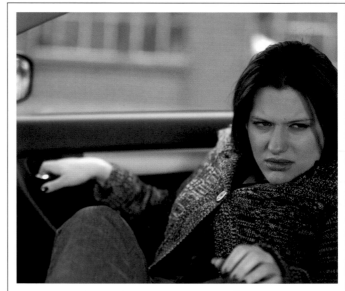

- Be prepared to make an exit at the first safe opportunity.

- Find the handle before you need it. Sometimes it can be hard to locate, and you'll need those critical seconds to make your escape when the time is right.

- Be careful not to pull the handle while the car is moving—especially if your back is against the door. Place your hand along the handle but wait for the right time to pull.

might choose to hug the shoulder strap or loop it partway around you.

If the driver is attacking you while driving the vehicle, you will need to make decisions about when it is appropriate to strike him. If the car is moving at extremely high speeds, it might risk your safety to make him lose control of the vehicle. In some cases, though, your best way to escape might be to cause the driver to crash. Weigh your options carefully against the severity of the situation. Remember that the overall goal is your safe escape from the situation. In the big picture, it does you no good to escape someone hitting you by injuring yourself in an automobile crash.

Seatbelts

- If you protect yourself as shown here, it is difficult to wear a seatbelt.

- At high speeds protection against accident may be the priority. At lower speeds it might be sufficient to hug the shoulder strap.

- In a moving vehicle, you must use your best judgment to decide which is the greater hazard: The assault or the possibility of a car accident.

- Keep in mind the big picture: Protecting yourself from all threats.

Escape When Safely Possible

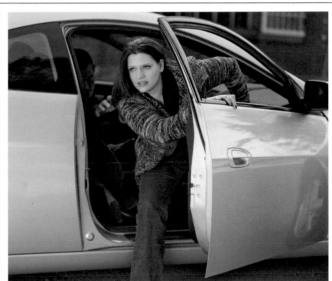

- As soon as the opportunity presents itself, pull the door handle and run from the vehicle.

- If possible, the safest choice will always be a time when the car has stopped.

- If doing this is not an option, you must use your best judgment. Decide if the risk of injury from bailing out at slow speeds is less than the risk of injury from waiting for a better opportunity.

- Do not wait to arrive at your destination.

189

ON AN AIRPLANE

Sometimes an environment dictates that exit is impossible

Self-defense on an airplane commonly comes up in questions. Although the probability of needing to engage in hand-to-hand combat on a commercial flight is tremendously low, many people ask this question as they consider terrorist situations and the like. Although it may not be a common situation, it has some factors that are worth discussing because they can happen in other environments as well.

First, airplanes are a good example of environments where

escape is not an option. You cannot elude your attacker by outrunning him or by getting away to a remote, safe location. You have an extremely limited environment in this regard.

Second, on an airplane you cannot rely on help from law enforcement or people who are more qualified to handle the situation than you are. Although other people may be present, you have no guarantee that they will be any better prepared for this than you. You must be empowered to do

On an Airplane

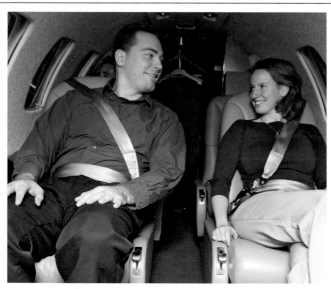

- Air travel is, as a rule, a very safe environment. It is highly unlikely that you will ever need to defend yourself during an airline flight.

- It is natural to be vigilant in this environment—you are surrounded by strangers in an enclosed space.

- While you should always remain aware of your environment, avoid excess paranoia. Be equally open to all possibilities—positive or negative. It isn't always necessary to be suspicious of others, unless their actions or behavior give reason for alarm.

The Space You Have

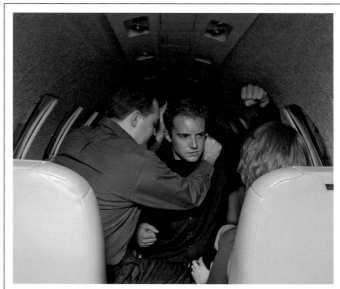

- On commercial airplanes you must engage your attacker in the limited space provided.

- Although you may have an opportunity to stand elsewhere, it is most likely you would have to confront him from your seat, or along the primary corridor.

- This kind of space makes surprise difficult. You must choose your timing carefully in order to catch him off guard.

- Be direct, aggressive, and overwhelming in your approach.

whatever you can to resolve this crisis. Take the initiative.

Third, an airplane has limited items in its environment. You must use what's at hand—which is preselected to eliminate most common weapons—to aid you.

Fourth, an air voyage cannot end the moment you deal with an attack. Your attacker will need to be restrained or otherwise incapacitated until the plane has time to land and the attacker can be transferred to the custody of the authorities.

Fifth, there are often many innocent bystanders on a commercial flight. If possible, you should do what you can to protect other people from the assailant. Many people may be at risk.

Finally, you may need to administer medical care to yourself or others following the assault. There is no guarantee that medically trained personnel will be present.

Use Your Environment

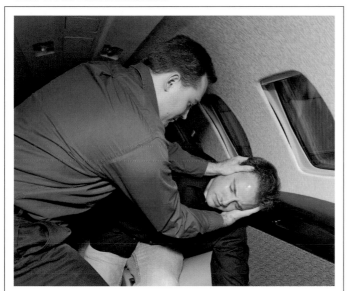

- Use the limited amount of space to maneuver as an advantage. It limits your attacker as much as it limits you.

- If there are solid objects nearby, use them as weapons. Drive him into the dividing wall between seating sections, the over- head bin, a nearby seat, a food cart, or anything else available.

- If you can, minimize the risk to other passengers. Move him away from them as you take control of the situation.

Enlist Help from Others

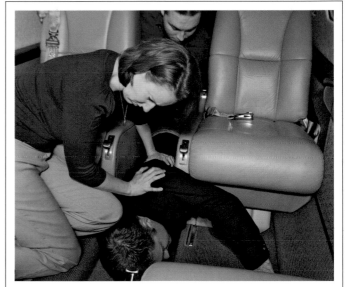

- Because there is no escape from this environment, you must ensure that the attacker presents no further threat until the plane has landed.

- Recruit others to assist you in immobilizing him. Some airliners carry restraint devices that can be used in these situations.

- If no restraint device is available to you, enlist several people to assist in holding the attacker until the plane has landed and help arrives.

ATTRACTING ATTENTION
Call others to your aid when a situation becomes violent

There is great debate in the self-defense industry over whether you should yell for help if you are being attacked.

The reason for the debate is this: In some communities calling for help might bring others to your aid. In other communities people might tend to avoid trouble and choose not to become involved, even if it's clear you need help. Sometimes instructors suggest yelling, "Fire!" or other similar alarms in the hope that they will attract others who wish to

be helpful but who might avoid entering a violent situation.

Try yelling, "Call 911!" instead of these other options. When people hear these instructions, they may choose to call as a way of helping indirectly without putting themselves in harm's way or inviting other consequences. It's not necessary that bystanders understand the nature of the emergency in order to summon aid; they can explain to the dispatcher that someone is yelling for help. They also have

Set Boundaries

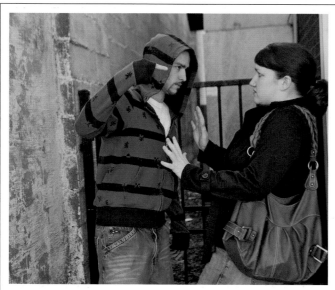

- When facing someone who may intend violence, set boundaries such as:

- "You are too close to me. Back off."

- "You are in my personal space. Move back."

- Speak in a loud, clear voice.

Doing this serves dual purposes: It firmly communicates your boundary to the aggressor, but it also calls attention to the inappropriate behavior.

- If others are watching or are within earshot, doing this makes the situation clear to everyone.

Describe the Problem

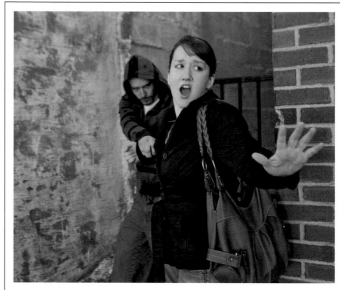

- If the situation continues, you can continue alerting others by describing the event:

- "Take your hands off of my arm."

- "That man took my purse."

- "I am not going anywhere with you. I don't know you."

- Speak loudly and clearly. Describe what's happening and what's inappropriate. Even if others can't see you (or can't see you well), describing the event will help bring them into the situation.

the luxury of explaining things in a calm and clear manner, which is not something you can do in the heat of an assault. By taking this objective out of your hands, it can be accomplished without delay—perhaps before your assault is fully realized or before you are able to escape.

No matter how you go about it, attract attention to yourself and your situation. Involve others as best you can. Summon any support that will make itself available to you, whether it comes in the form of trained professionals or just passers-by. The more people you have on your side, the better the odds in your favor. Try to recruit others in the hopes that they will intercede.

"Call 911!"

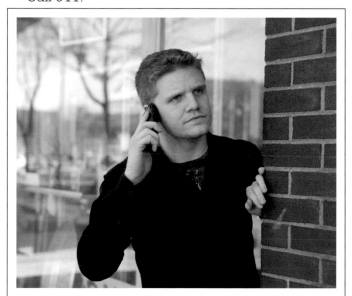

- If you need help, one reliable alarm to yell is "Call 911!"

- Although some bystanders will be hesitant to become involved personally, calling for emergency assistance is something a person can do to help that will not put him in harm's way.

- Even if the person is unclear on what's happening, by calling 911 he brings aid to the scene. In a crisis this is immensely valuable.

Whistles and Sirens

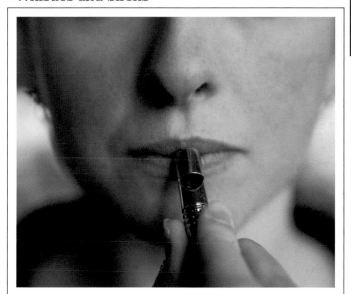

- From whistles and alarms to sirens and miniature air horns, many varieties of personal noisemakers are available to help you attract attention.

- Some devices are activated by pulling out a pin or key, after which they will continue making noises of up to 130 decibels (approximately the volume of an airplane, rock concert, or ambulance siren).

- Devices that create this level of noise can also cause injury if deployed near your assailant's face.

CALLING 911
If you're able to call for help, be prepared to give the right info

Calls to 911 can be placed before, during, or after an assault takes place. Each of these times may take a different approach and will bring about different resolution.

Calling 911 prior to the full height of the crisis may seem the most difficult because the assault hasn't happened yet. In some situations it may seem that the call is not warranted—for example, if someone threatens you but has not yet acted out physically. You may not be entirely comfortable calling

at this stage of events, but it's important to remember that intervening at this early time may prevent the crisis from evolving further.

A more common application of preassault contact with emergency services might be coming home to find that someone has broken into your home. Rather than entering the house, you should move a safe distance away and call 911. If the perpetrators are still inside, you could walk into

Safe Opportunity to Call

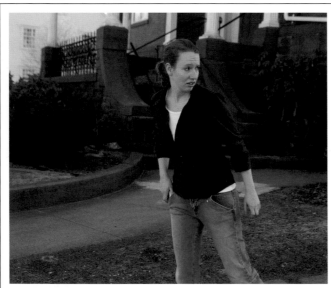

- If you are calling from a cell phone, be prepared to reach an operator who will ask the nature of your emergency and the city you're calling from. The operator will then reroute your call to a local operator who can dispatch aid to you.

- 911 operators will typically ask for a callback number in the event you are disconnected. If you cannot provide one, remember that you will need to call back if the call is interrupted.

"What Is Your Location?"

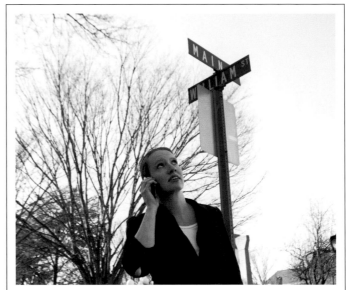

- The first question an operator will ask you is for your exact location. The more precisely you can identify your whereabouts, the more effectively help will reach you.

- Identify a nearby street address or intersection. If you cannot locate a sign,

find a landmark that can help identify your location.

- Be as specific as possible. If you are indoors, identify the floor and the suite, office, or room. If you are outside, tell the operator where you are relative to the address you've identified.

harm's way by entering. Have law enforcement clear the building first.

During an assault, it is unlikely that the victim (whether it's you or someone else) will be the person calling 911, although it can happen. Your real priority in that moment, if you are under attack, is to protect yourself. Create safety for yourself by getting away or neutralizing the attack before focusing on the call for support.

After an assault has occurred, placing a call to 911 is one of the most important steps in transitioning into your postcrisis management plan. It is done to make sure that your safety is maintained—you are no longer in danger, and things will stay that way after support arrives to assist you.

Call 911 even if the crisis appears to be resolved. If there are future legal or medical consequences, you will want as much documentation to support you as you can gather.

"Are You Hurt?"

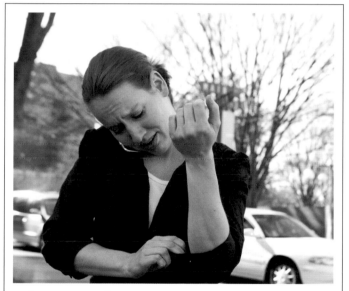

- If you are injured, you will need the dispatcher to send medical assistance.

- Evaluate yourself as you talk with the operator. Check yourself for injury as best you can. Evaluate your arms, legs, torso, and head.

- If you were hit during the attack or have fallen down, check for any blood or open cuts. Check fingers and toes for breaks or dislocations. Evaluate your neck for any kind of spinal injury.

Stay on the Line

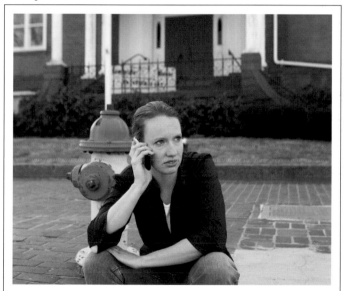

- If it is safe to do so, the operator will often ask you to stay on the line until help arrives to assist you.

- If your location is safe, stay there. You want it to be as easy as possible for aid to reach you.

- The operator may have additional questions for you. He or she will also be able to help you if trouble reappears or if you suddenly need medical attention.

ASSESSING EXITS
In a crisis every option you have is a powerful asset

Finding and evaluating your exit options are critical in any kind of crisis situation. Most of us are creatures of habit and notice only the primary entrances and exits. When the chips are down, you want to have as many options as possible. Note the exits and evaluate them according to the following features:

First: Where are the primary exits? Where are the doors for the public, for the staff, and for emergencies? Where does each of these lead? Do you know where these will open out to, or will you need to find your way after you pass through them?

Second: Where are the secondary exits? Are there windows you can use? Are there stairs or ladders to other paths that will take you away from this situation? If you are indoors, what floor are you on? What floors feature exits?

Third: Are any of these exits unsafe? Are there hazards surrounding them? Is there fire, electricity, traffic, heights, or broken glass?

Buildings Have Many Exits

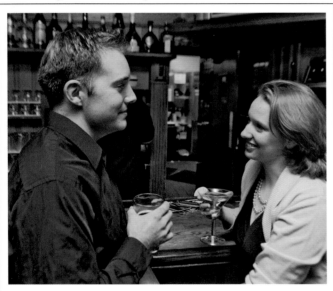

- We have all been conditioned by routine to enter and exit restaurants, stores, and the other places we go via the public exit.

- Most commercial storefronts offer one to two primary doors, and yet they have numerous other points of entry or exit for staff members and for deliveries.

- In a crisis situation, the nearest exit may not be an obvious one. It may be through the kitchen or a "staff only" door. It may be out through a back office, warehouse, or loading dock.

Broken Exit

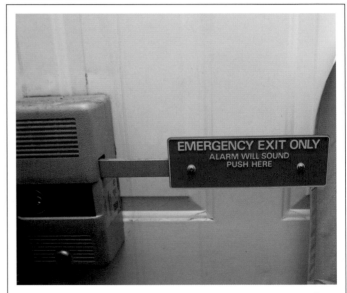

- Sometimes a path that should be available isn't. There may be construction, renovations, faulty equipment, or a host of other blockages of that route.

- Look for multiple points of exit in case one is unavailable to you.

- In some cases it may still be possible to exit through a construction area or a broken exit. But be careful and watch your step—most likely, it was blocked off for a good reason, and you need to be aware of safety risks.

Fourth: Can you reach the exit? Are there obstacles that make it difficult or impossible to make use of that exit? Is a crowd of people blocking your way? Is there construction? A fence? A wall?

Last: Where are you going? Are you simply running away from trouble, or are you running toward your destination? Where should your destination be? Is there a vehicle you can use to bring yourself farther away? Do you have keys or access to public transportation?

Make yourself aware of the exits when you enter a new environment. Don't be paranoid or worry about them; simply be observant and take note. Have you lived or worked in an environment like this one? Can you guess, from experience, what the rest of the building is like and where the exits may be?

Blocked Exits

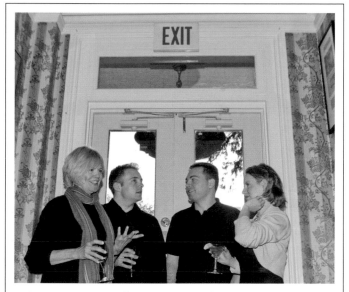

- Sometimes it's not the exit itself that presents difficulty but rather the act of reaching it.

- There may be crowds of people, objects, or safety hazards between you and the exit.

- In these cases it may be necessary to find a secondary exit that doesn't present the same difficulties. Scout the room for other options.

- Dense crowds of people can be one of the toughest environments to navigate. Weigh your options as you choose your exit.

Emergency Exit

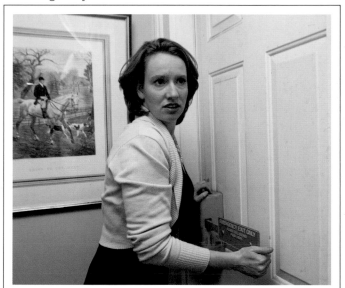

- Most of us endure so few crisis situations that we start to ignore emergency exits because we never need them.

- Many emergency exits are alarmed, which can benefit you in a crisis; some alarms will send security or police to your location.

- Take a step back and remind yourself where the emergency exits are in the places you frequent.

- It sometimes takes a moment to remember that these crisis situations are the exact thing for which those exits are created: Emergencies.

197

GETTING AWAY
Put space between yourself and your assailant until you can find help

One of the least examined moments in self-defense training is the moment of running away. It receives constant attention in a broad way: We discuss its importance and when to do it. We remind everyone that it is the top priority and that we should practice distancing ourselves from our attacker in our hands-on training. But what are the keys to getting away safely?

Certain skills play a critical role. First and foremost, you need to be able to run. The farther and faster your running will take you, the better. When it comes to running, what is your current fitness level? Are you more suited for short distances or long ones? Are you better with long straight-aways or quick changes of direction?

Create Your Opportunity

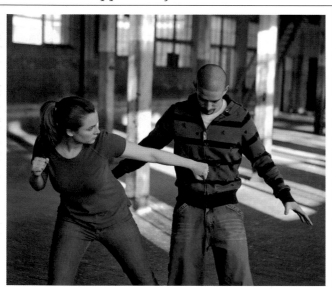

- In situations where escaping is a possibility, look for the first sign that you have time enough to get away.

- Sometimes you can land a good strike and see the opportunity to flee. Do not hesitate if that moment appears: Go.

- The most important skill in your initial escape is your ability to run. Know your own capabilities: How long can you sprint? At what speed? How far will that take you? What if someone is chasing you?

Navigate Obstacles

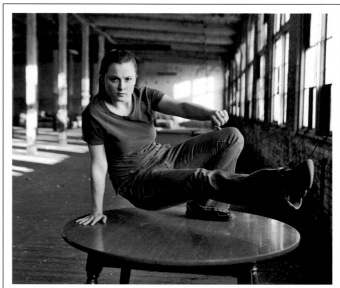

- In moving toward your escape, it may be necessary to traverse obstacles in your environment.

- If you have the skill or ability to jump, hurdle, climb, or otherwise navigate over and around obstacles that others may find difficult,

  this is a valuable tool in your exit.

- If the most direct route to the exit involves going over (or under) a nearby table or other obstacle, give it a look. It may buy you valuable seconds (and distance) as you put your attacker behind you.

Second, you may need the ability to climb. How high an object can you climb over? Can you climb a wall? A tree? A telephone pole? Could you enter the second story of a house from the outside if you absolutely had to? What about a building or a parking garage? How quickly can you climb?

Third, you may need the ability to jump. How high can you jump if you need to reach something? How far can you jump if you have to traverse a gap? Can you land on something narrow? Something rounded? Something moving?

Fourth, can you swim? Are you a strong or fast swimmer?

Can you swim or tread water for long periods of time if necessary? How long can you swim underwater without surfacing to take a breath?

People with backgrounds in running, gymnastics, rock climbing, parkour, and traversing obstacle courses will have certain advantages when it comes to making an escape. What skills do you have when it comes to getting away? What are your strengths and weaknesses in this arena?

Locate the Right Path

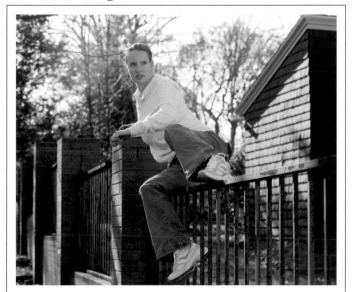

- In picking your escape path, take into account any specific knowledge you may have of the area or any personal abilities or training you have.

- People who are experienced gymnasts, runners, climbers, traceurs, acrobats, and the like may be able to follow routes that the average person cannot.

- If you know the area well, you may be aware of particular paths that are not obvious but that give you an advantage for escape or hiding.

Find Help

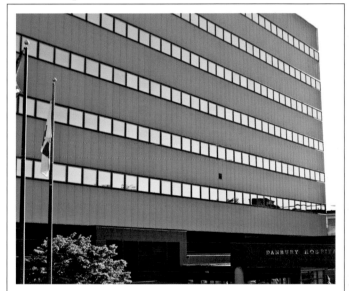

- The best thing to find when escaping an assault is a place where help is available.

- Although police and fire stations may be the most obvious, many other destinations offer security personnel, including hospitals, corporate buildings, shopping malls, and banks.

- If in making your escape you come upon a place that has trained staff who can help you, you may find sanctuary in the hands of these professionals.

WHEN TO STOP HITTING
If you're able to get the upper hand, when should you stop?

In an ideal hands-on situation, you are able to establish the advantage in the conflict and neutralize the attack by physically defeating your assailant. How do you know when this has occurred?

First and foremost, you look for indications that your attacker is no longer willing or able to continue the assault. Inability can manifest itself in a severe injury or unconsciousness. Unwillingness is demonstrated in body language—most

notably, the cessation of any physical or verbal hostilities in the direction of you or any other intended victims. If you encounter these indicators, use your best judgment to evaluate their authenticity. If you conclude that they are genuine, you can halt your counterattack safely.

In this decision you must err on the side of caution. It is reasonable to assume that the attack is continuing until you have concrete evidence to the contrary. To assume otherwise

Attacker Assumes Fetal Position

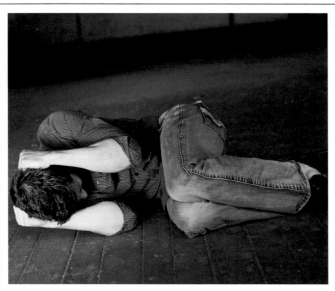

- One sign that the attacker no longer wishes to continue the assault is a fetal position.

- If he curls into a ball to weather your strikes, it is a sign that he is retreating from his intended assault.

- Use your best judgment to determine if he is only protecting himself for a second or if he is no longer interested in continuing his attack.

Attacker Is Unconscious

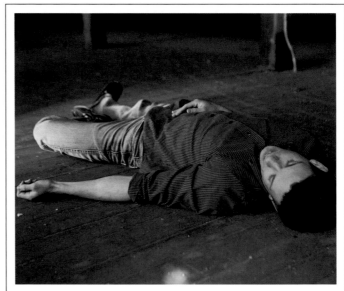

- If your attacker goes unconscious, this is a clear sign that you have regained safety, at least for a time, and that it is no longer necessary to continue striking him.

- Depending on the situation, this may be your opportunity to run away or

to find a way to restrain him before he awakens.

- If law enforcement or other help has been summoned, his unconsciousness will keep him at bay for a time while you wait for help to arrive and more fully restrain him.

would expose you to unnecessary risk if you mistakenly judge him "finished" and he is still intent on doing you harm. You should maintain the advantage until you are absolutely clear that your safety is assured.

Because this decision involves judgment, it is possible that it will open you up to consequences later. There may be legal or ethical questions about whether you overstepped your rights in defending yourself. It's important in these cases to be able to analyze the decisions you made, especially the decision to start fighting back and the decision to cease fighting. If you can clearly explain the factors that you evaluated in making these decisions—defining his actions that showed aggression and violent intent and his later actions that showed he was no longer pursuing the attack—then you should find yourself covered in most arenas.

Attacker Is Injured

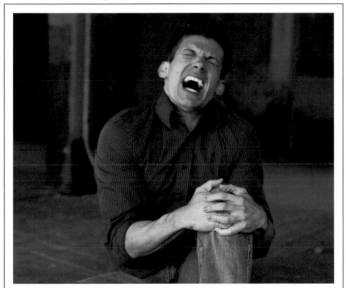

- If your attacker sustains a serious injury, this may be an opportunity for you to stop defending yourself and to run.

- In particular, if he is unable to chase you, then most threats will end at this point.

- Depending on the severity of the injury, it may buy you a small window of opportunity or a much larger one.

- Use your best judgment to ascertain the extent of his injury and how much it is impairing him.

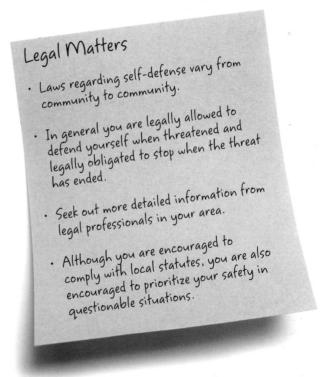

Legal Matters

- Laws regarding self-defense vary from community to community.

- In general you are legally allowed to defend yourself when threatened and legally obligated to stop when the threat has ended.

- Seek out more detailed information from legal professionals in your area.

- Although you are encouraged to comply with local statutes, you are also encouraged to prioritize your safety in questionable situations.

MINIMIZING INJURY

If you're losing the fight, how can you protect yourself from serious injury?

Although it's a difficult topic, you must consider the possibility that despite your best efforts, you may come out on the losing end of the altercation. It's time to look at the big picture and how you can manage this possibility.

If you find yourself overwhelmed and unable to escape, you need to take steps to protect yourself so that you are not injured severely. Curl into a small shape and protect your head and torso with your arms and legs. You want to prevent injury to the brain and major organs. An injury to an arm or a leg heals much more quickly than severe internal injury, and it is much less likely to be life threatening.

If you can, use your environment by placing yourself against

Covering Your Head

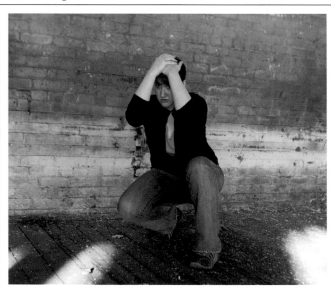

- The most natural response if you're taking blows is to protect your head. This should be encouraged.

- You want to protect the face from injury because many of the bones are delicate. You also want to protect the eyes, which are particularly vulnerable.

- Head injury can be a serious matter, so you want to absorb as much as you can on your arms rather than your head.

"Turtled" Up

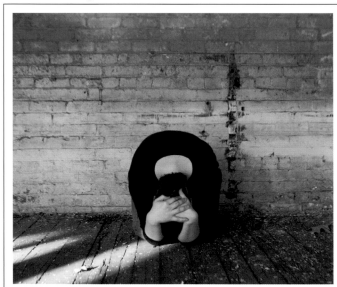

- In severe situations you can "turtle up" into a ball on the ground.

- This is done to protect the face, head, and internal organs.

- The body is curled around the torso, with the knees and elbows tucked. The

- forearms protect the face, which is turned toward the ground or against one arm.

- Shield your body from the most vicious blows. Be aware that your spine is still vulnerable in this position but that your major organs are protected.

a wall or another solid object that can protect you on one or more sides. If you can crawl under a table or other shelter, you may be able to lessen the extent of your injuries.

At a certain point, a decision needs to be made about whether you improve or worsen the consequences by fighting back. In some situations it will be appropriate to fight until you absolutely cannot fight anymore. In other situations you may find it prudent to change to a defensive approach sooner rather than later. No matter the choice, any of these situations will have a range of physical and emotional

consequences to manage afterward. Knowing yourself and your own constitution can go a long way toward making the best decision you can in these tough situations.

These are not pleasant decisions by any stretch of the imagination; however, they are possible scenarios that you should consider as you prepare yourself for the best and worst possible situations.

Back against a Wall

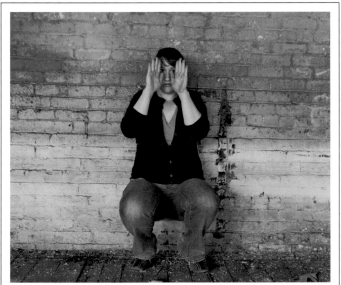

- If you can, use a wall or other obstacle to provide protection on one side.

- Back yourself against it or curl up in front of it to provide a small amount of shielding.

- As before, use your knees and forearms to cover your body. Protect the face and internal organs as best you can. Keep attacks away from your eyes, groin, and other sensitive areas to minimize pain.

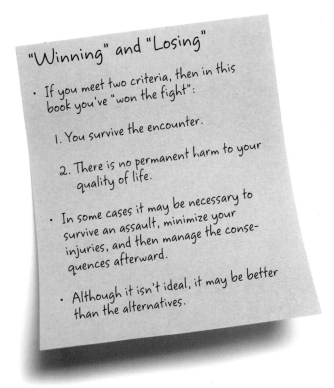

"Winning" and "Losing"

- If you meet two criteria, then in this book you've "won the fight":

  1. You survive the encounter.

  2. There is no permanent harm to your quality of life.

- In some cases it may be necessary to survive an assault, minimize your injuries, and then manage the consequences afterward.

- Although it isn't ideal, it may be better than the alternatives.

IS THERE STILL DANGER?

Your first priority is to be sure that you are safe and that the danger has passed

Prioritize your postassault care into several issues. The first and most important issue is whether you are still in danger. The support structure you need, if danger persists, will come from law enforcement.

The most critical aid that law enforcement officers (LEOs) can provide is a buffer of safety between you and your assailant. Whether he is still attempting to attack you or you fear that he may resume his attack later, LEOs can provide you with protection in the immediate moment and take your attacker into custody.

LEOs are trained and armed with a bevy of skills and tools that allows them to assist you. They are also well networked

Are You in Danger?

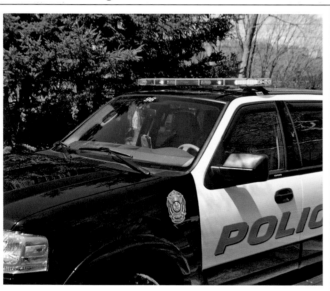

- The most critical step in ending an assault is finding a safe environment.

- Your first priority is to make sure that the assault is over. If the attacker pursues you personally, you will need either to finish the fight or to enlist help from those who can.

- When in doubt, recruit aid. You want to be sure that the attack will not continue when you let down your guard.

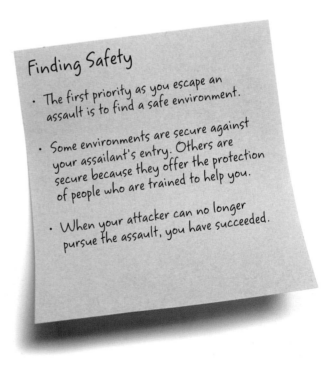

Finding Safety

- The first priority as you escape an assault is to find a safe environment.

- Some environments are secure against your assailant's entry. Others are secure because they offer the protection of people who are trained to help you.

- When your attacker can no longer pursue the assault, you have succeeded.

with other forms of support and can summon medical aid or offer transportation to you.

Confirming that the attack is over and that you are now safe is a major priority. This confirmation will be critical to your ability to receive adequate care both immediately after the attack and in the long term. Do not skip this priority and assume that all is well. Recruit aid and see to it that you are well protected.

Law Enforcement Officers

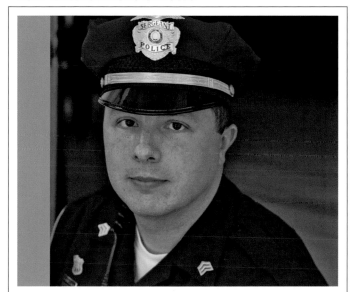

- Law enforcement officers should be your first line of protection because they offer the tools and skills to end the threat to your safety.

- LEOs are trained to help protect you from an attack. Involve them as quickly as possible if you are still under threat.

- Even if the assault is over, you will need the help of LEOs to prevent a recurrence of the attack.

Removing the Assailant

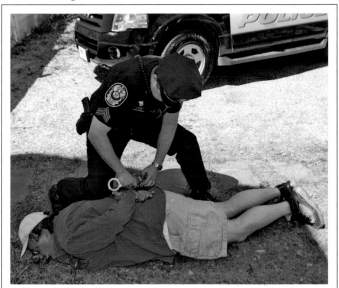

- At the very least, law enforcement officers can act as a buffer between your assailant and you.

- They can prevent the attack from continuing by restraining him or removing him from the scene.

- Arresting the attacker is also the first step in preventing a second assault at a later time.

- LEOs can also help provide you with resources to begin your postassault management. They can connect you with medical attention, lawyers, and the like.

ARE YOU HURT?

When the crisis is over, the next priority is to receive medical treatment for any injuries

The second priority of postassault management should be to identify and treat any injuries or health risks. To do this you will need quality medical care.

In most cases immediate medical treatment involves two phases: An emergency responder of some kind will initially evaluate and treat you on scene, and then you will be brought to the local emergency room to receive further care.

At the initial scene, you may be treated by an EMT, paramedic, firefighter, or first responder. Their job is to assess your injuries and ensure that you are stable for the journey to the hospital.

After you arrive at the emergency room, you will again be

Are You Injured?

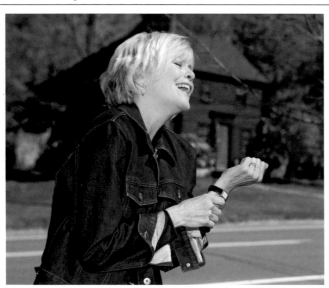

- It is quite likely that you sustained an injury of some kind either during the assault or during your escape.

- Because you will undoubtedly be adrenalized by the experience, you may not realize you've been injured until much later.

- When you reach safety, check yourself for blood, tender or painful areas, or any sprains or broken bones.

- Sometimes injuries will not present themselves until later. Seek medical treatment as soon as possible to avoid complications.

Seek Medical Aid

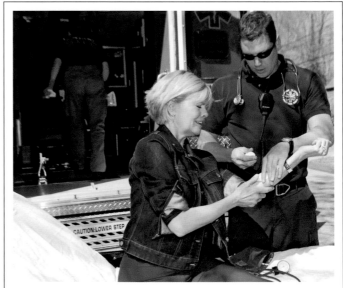

- If you have just survived an assault, you should seek medical aid to be checked for injuries.

- Many injuries, especially head wounds, may not be apparent to you. Have yourself examined to be sure that you haven't missed any injuries or traumas.

- Put yourself into the hands of professionals to be sure that your attack won't have further medical repercussions.

- Even if they find nothing, it is much better to be sure than to find a serious condition later.

evaluated, this time by doctors or nurses. They may discharge you if your injuries are insignificant; they may treat you; or they may refer you to another doctor for further care.

If you have any broken bones, you will likely see an orthopedist and have some X-rays taken. If there is evidence of trauma to your head, you may be sent to a neurologist or be administered a CT scan. If you have been through a sexual assault—or don't know whether you have been sexually assaulted—medical workers will often send you to an OB/GYN for consultation and evaluation for evidence of assault.

Self-administering Medical Aid

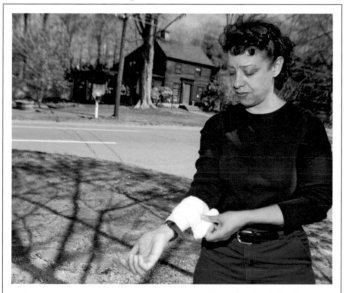

- In some cases you may need to self-administer medical treatment. If you sustain a serious injury, you might need to treat it while you wait for medical professionals to reach you.

- Seek out training in basic first aid so that you can learn to identify conditions such as shock, dehydration, and more. You will also learn to bandage, cover, or splint basic injuries.

- You may want to keep basic first aid supplies in easy-to-access locations such as your purse or the glove compartment in your vehicle.

Treating Your Companions

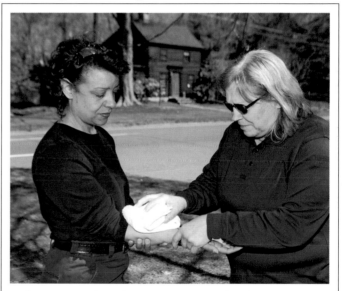

- If you are not the only victim of the attack, it may be necessary to treat others' injuries as well.

- While you await medical professionals, examine your companions and have them check you. Look for obvious injuries such as cuts, bruises, and broken bones.

- First aid and CPR training are available in most communities and fairly inexpensively. It can be a worthwhile investment, even if you use it only once. The time it saves you and your loved ones in a crisis could be critical.

POSTCRISIS MANAGEMENT

GIVING A STATEMENT

Most situations will require you to record a statement with law enforcement officers

In almost any attack law enforcement will become involved. One of the steps you should be prepared for is the process of giving a statement to the officers who respond. This preparation is the third step of postassault management.

To help facilitate this step of the process, you should select a friend whom you can call at any hour in a crisis. It helps if the friend has an alpha male-type personality, but it is not absolutely necessary.

After ensuring your safety and receiving necessary medical attention, call the friend and instruct him to come help you. His job will be to act as your agent with the officer who will take your statement and to make sure that you have

KNACK SELF-DEFENSE FOR WOMEN

Talk with Your Friend

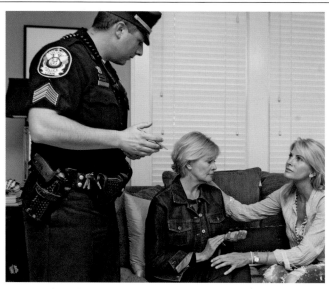

- Your friend's job is to make sure that you are given the time to calm down in order to make your statement.

- You can talk things over with your friend. It's a good idea to rehash the events in order to straighten them out in your mind.

- Your friend can help by listening to you, asking questions, and helping to calm you. You'll need to be calm and rational before giving a statement.

Take the Necessary Time

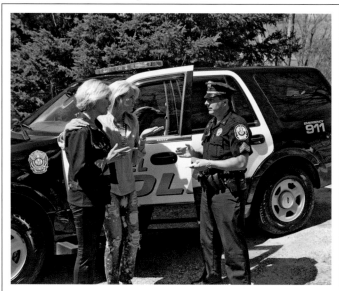

- If law enforcement is already on the scene, your friend can act as your agent and let the officers know how much time you will need before making your statement.

- If the police have not yet been notified, and you do not need medical attention, your friend can be the person who calls to alert them and to tell them how long to wait before coming to take your statement.

adequate time to calm down and compose yourself and your thoughts before you give your statement.

You can even give him a script to follow, along the lines of "Officer, thanks so much for coming. My friend is obviously shaken up, and she'll be ready to give a statement in a couple hours." Your friend should be polite but firm in assuring that you have sufficient time to prepare yourself to be accurate in describing what happened.

If law enforcement officers have not yet been called, your friend can also be the person who contacts them. "My friend has been attacked. She has received appropriate medical care and will need an officer to come in a couple of hours to take a statement."

The reason for taking such deliberate steps to calm you before you give a statement is that your words are recorded as though this was your calmest, most rational moment. The officer acts in this duty as an officer of the court and records this document for legal use later. It is critical that you are as accurate as possible and do not distort events (whether intentionally or not).

Making Your Statement

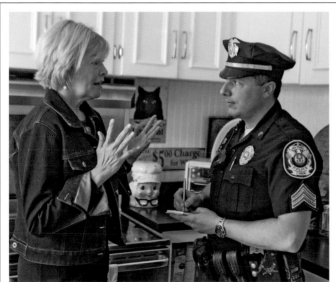

- Give yourself adequate time to prepare before making your statement. You want to be sure that you are as accurate as possible.

- In taking your statement, the officer is acting as an officer of the court. He is tasked with recording your statement exactly, so that it can be used in legal proceedings later.

- Details will be scrutinized at later times. Be sure that you've calmed yourself adequately and can express clearly what happened.

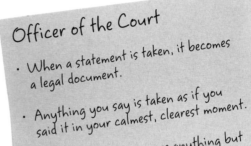

Officer of the Court

- When a statement is taken, it becomes a legal document.

- Anything you say is taken as if you said it in your calmest, clearest moment.

- After an assault you are anything but calm. You may unintentionally distort the facts or misremember events while you are agitated.

- Take the time you need to prepare before making your statement. Accuracy is extremely valuable.

LEGAL HELP
Protecting yourself continues after the assault is over

The fourth step of postassault management is to secure appropriate legal support. You must protect yourself legally against any consequences that arise from the attack. There are a few consequences that you may face as a result of the assault. In today's world legal consequences can arise in even the most nonsensical situations. In some cases an attacker may assault you just to sue you afterward. Although this may sound laughable, the phenomenon (and others

like it) does happen. It's important that just as you protect yourself physically from harm, you must also protect yourself from legal aftereffects.

The types of legal consequences, both criminal and civil, that can emerge from an assault vary widely from region to region, as do the processes that govern them. Find out about the laws in your area to avoid surprises.

Legal affairs can drag on for an extended period of time. It

Criminal Actions

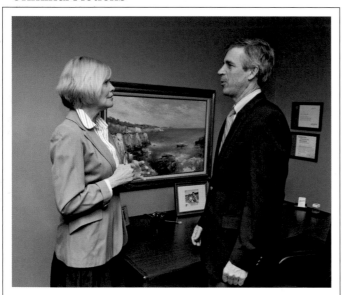

- The first type of legal action you may encounter after an assault is criminal charges.

- You may make charges against your attacker, or there may be charges against you.

- Some women are hesitant to press charges against

their attackers. Sometimes they feel that doing so only prolongs the emotional trauma of the attack.

- It is recommended that you pursue the criminal charges, if for no other reason than to prevent future assaults—against you or against others.

Civil Actions

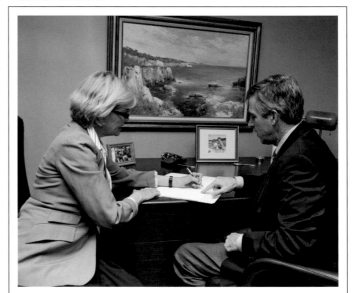

- The second kind of action you may face is civil litigation, which is more commonly known as a "lawsuit."

- Civil actions occur when one person seeks reparations (typically money) from another person as a result of some damages.

- It may be that you are pressing a suit against your attacker, or your attacker may press a suit against you.

- A third party might also claim damages as a result of the assault and name you as a participant.

may be difficult to continue rehashing the assault, and also it may cause you emotional and financial hardship to do so. Finding a good lawyer who can advise you about all of the ramifications, including their upsides and downsides, is absolutely essential.

Order of Protection

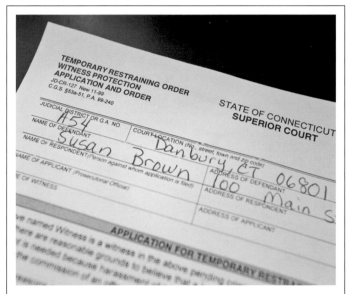

- Protective orders are legal injunctions that forbid someone from coming within a certain distance of you or of select locations such as your home or workplace.

- Laws regarding protective orders vary from state to state. Depending on the local laws, they may be filed in criminal court, civil court, or both.

- Some protective orders also involve consequences for the perpetrator, including counseling or the surrender of firearms.

Courtroom Proceedings

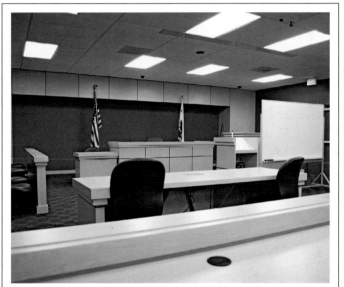

- Depending on the extent of the assault, legal proceedings may continue for some time.

- In some kinds of cases, you may need to retain legal counsel throughout. A variety of options (and price tags) may be available to you.

- Although it can be emotionally (and even financially) difficult to have prolonged interactions with your attacker via the justice system, the rewards are often well worth it.

YOUR CONTINUED WELL-BEING

It's important to keep tabs on your mental, physical, and emotional health after any crisis

The fifth and final step of your postassault management is to find support for your mental, physical, and emotional well-being as you move forward after the attack. You may experience a number of lasting consequences as a result of the assault, and it is important to seek assistance so that you can avoid permanent or severe consequences wherever possible.

Crisis events can change the landscape of your life. If you are lucky, you will not suffer any permanent harm to your quality of life—but the nature of your life may change considerably as a reaction to what has happened.

Draw upon the support of others as you come to terms with what has happened and the consequences that have arisen

Support from Your Family

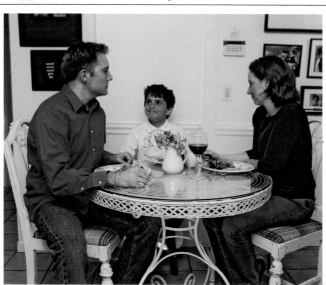

- The first support that you can and should draw upon is the security and emotional comfort of your loved ones.

- Friends and family are crucial to your postcrisis recovery because they can help you to sort through difficult emotions regard-

ing both the assault and its consequences.

- Take heed of their love and encouragement as you work to sustain your well-being and to work through any challenges that emerge.

Visit a Therapist

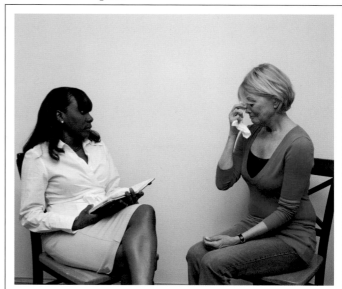

- Visiting a counselor can help you work through some of the emotional repercussions of the attack.

- Whether you visit a social worker, counselor, psychologist or psychiatrist, find someone who can help you attend to your mental and emotional needs.

- Some people will suffer from paranoia, post-traumatic stress disorder, depression, anxiety, and a host of other conditions after a violent assault.

- These conditions may emerge right away or over time. Seek help to manage them.

from it. Close ties with friends and family can be invaluable during this time. You may suffer from personality changes or strong emotional reactions to what has happened. Take comfort in the loyalty and friendship of loved ones.

Likewise, you may have ongoing medical issues as a result of the assault. These can be physical problems, mental health problems, or a mix of the two. Be sure to pursue treatment for any conditions that emerge.

Ongoing Medical Treatment

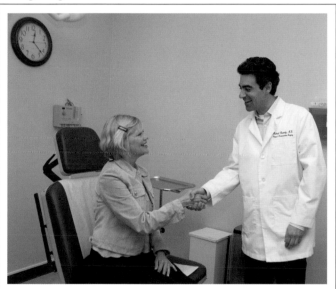

- In most cases immediate medical treatment will come from rescue workers, followed by your local emergency room.

- Depending on the nature of your assault, you may be sent to specialists or to your primary care physician for further treatment.

- You may be sent to an orthopedist for broken bones, or in cases of sexual assault you may be referred to an OB/GYN to deal with sexually transmitted infections or pregnancy.

Support Group Meetings

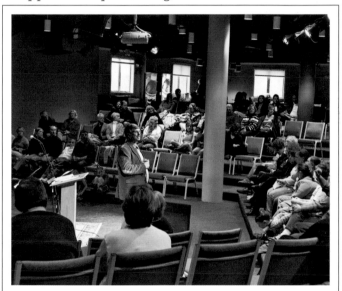

- Another source of comfort can be meetings with support groups.

- These are events for small groups of people who discuss their experiences and draw encouragement from each other as they manage the repercussions.

- Many support groups exist for people who have survived assaults, and they range in scope from general to specific. There are also many support groups and hotlines for depression, anxiety, and suicide. All of these can be valuable resources, depending on your needs.

ASSEMBLE YOUR TEAM NOW

Do the work before a crisis to make things easier when you need help

The hardest time to assemble your support team is immediately after an assault. You will be inundated with responsibilities, consequences, and options to evaluate. All of that makes this a terrible time for you to be searching the Internet or the local directory for a good lawyer, doctor, or therapist. Put together your team when things are at their best because that is the time when you can take your time to make the right choices.

Examine your situation closely and determine the people you will need on your team. Although it has been recommended that you find a good doctor, lawyer, therapist, and close friend, you may find that you need to add or delete

Connect with Professionals

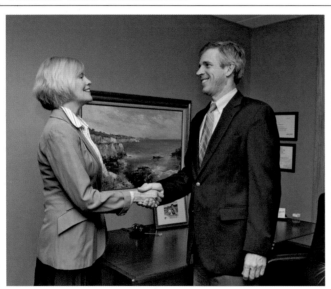

- Develop relationships with professionals who can help you during or after crisis situations.

- Talk with family and friends to get recommendations for doctors, lawyers, therapists, and so on. Meet people and evaluate their services when all is well.

- It rarely hurts to check in with these people while times are good. They can often help you bolster your protection against difficult consequences later.

- The better your relationship, the more you can rely upon their support when you most need it.

Store Contact Information

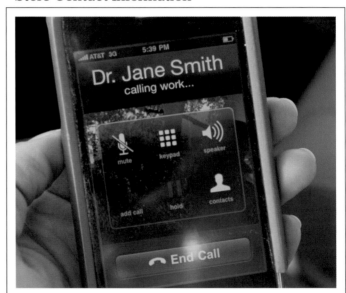

- Maintain access to these people by storing their contact information in a few places.

- First, store their phone numbers in your cell phone. That way you can reach them in a crisis.

- Next, keep hard copies of their information on file at home. This way, if you lose your phone, you can replace the information easily.

- Keep contact with them routinely. It can be helpful to you if they know you and know your situation.

members from that list. Perhaps you need a bodyguard, security consultant, or a personal assistant as part of your personal safety plan. If you know members of your local law enforcement community, they can be valuable assets. Decide what avenues you will need managed for you in a crisis and develop a support team that matches your needs.

MAKE IT EASY

Although we focused on postassault management, you can also assemble a team for any preassault steps you take. If you bring in professionals to fortify your home, teach you new skills, or evaluate your personal safety level, you can create a second, overlapping network of support. You may decide to improve your fitness level, employ a home security company, train in martial arts, or learn to fire a weapon.

Assemble Your Team

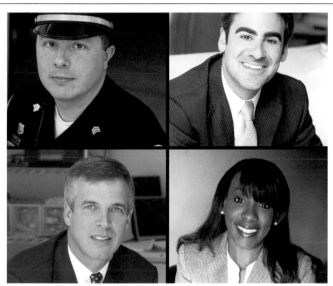

- Cover your bases before you find yourself in crisis. The last thing you need is to be in the middle of a turbulent situation and to add the stress of trying to find a good lawyer (or doctor or therapist).

- This list is by no means exhaustive. For you support may include team members we haven't mentioned, including personal assistants, bodyguards, and so on.

- Evaluate your situation and find people who match your needs.

Surround Yourself with Support

- The better prepared you can be, the greater your odds of preserving your quality of life if you endure an assault.

- Build up networks of supporting people, be they family, friends, or professionals.

- Help give yourself the tools to live a happy life and to manage turbulent events that occur along the way.

- Be proactive. It will be easier if you don't wait until you desperately need help.

SELF-DEFENSE WORKSHOPS
Short-term commitments for introductory skills

Hands-on skills are not a reasonable option for everyone. Although many women can derive tremendous benefit from the information and skills demonstrated in self-defense classes, such classes will not always be appropriate for you and your personal situation.

If you're not sure if hands-on training should be a part of your approach, look for a low-commitment opportunity to try it out and see what you think.

Self-defense workshops can be a great way to determine how (and how much) you will benefit from doing some training. They allow you to see how you feel as a student and to audition various instructors as a resource.

Self-defense workshops vary greatly, and the nature of the content relies entirely on the background of the instructor teaching. Many instructors in the martial arts and self-defense industry know little beyond their own chosen style

Finding Self-defense Workshops

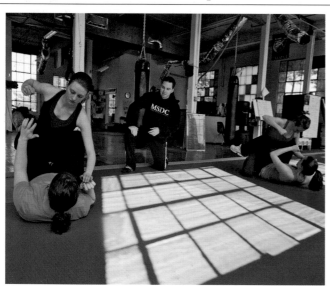

- Most people have access to self-defense workshops in their local area.

- Workshops are a good short-term solution for people who have limited time or money or who want only a little exposure to see if hands-on training is appropriate for them.

- If you have trouble finding a workshop, check out college campuses or talk to local law enforcement. They can often put you in contact with instructors.

- Workshops may meet only once or for several weeks in a row.

Immediate Needs

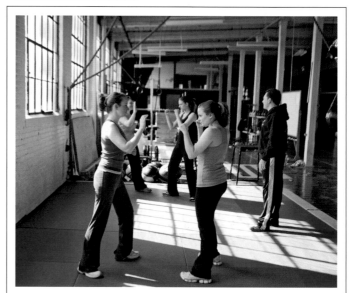

- Most self-defense workshops focus on skills that are quickly learned and broadly useful.

- The most important skills revolve around identification and prevention in the preassault stage. Some workshops focus exclusively

- on these aspects without even offering a hands-on portion.

- Other workshops will focus entirely on physical responses. Most will show simple, easily learned skills that should be appropriate for all body types.

and may lack much (or any) experience using what they teach. Unfortunately there are few ways to determine ahead of time whether an instructor will present useful information—especially information that is useful to you.

If you are looking for a low-cost, short-term way of checking out some training, try attending some self-defense workshops, ideally taught by different instructors from different arts, styles, or organizations. Find a group or an instructor whose perspective aligns with your own. If you trust their judgment, let them guide you in determining the options that will be worth your time to pursue. Instructors run a wide gamut, so keep searching until you find one who meets your needs. Or, if after several attempts, you cannot find instruction that is meaningful to you, explore other options beyond martial arts and self-defense training.

Specialty Workshops

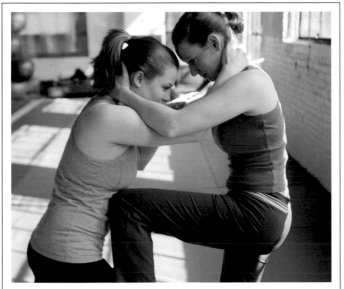

- Most workshops will have a particular focus or theme. Depending on the type of instructor, you may learn any of a broad variety of skills.

- There are no overarching organizations that run the self-defense industry, so there is no guarantee that the information will be relevant to you.

- Do your homework ahead of time and learn the teachers' specialty. Find out their credentials and see if they sound right for you.

Workshops Can Offer Value

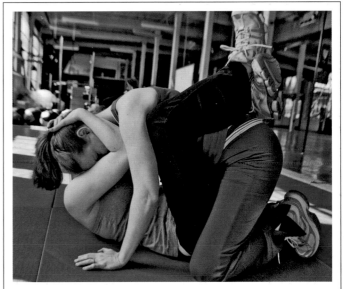

- A good workshop will help you identify risk factors in your own life and provide you with reasonable options to help improve your safety while maintaining your quality of life.

- The advantage of workshops is that they typically require little commitment on your part in regard to both your time and your money.

- They can offer you the opportunity to learn valuable skills and to "test drive" instructions from instructors in your community if you are considering seeking further training.

KRAV MAGA

Israeli combatives are a great route for quick skills and killer instinct

Krav Maga is a modern system of combatives that originated within the Israeli military. It is now available to military, law enforcement, and civilians (in slightly different forms).

By design Krav Maga is intended to be learned in a short period of time and retained well with minimal practice. It employs a small but deep curriculum of well-planned, natural movements that is vicious and aggressive.

Krav Maga training acknowledges that in real combat there are no rules and that thus its practitioners should be ready for anything. It attacks the most vulnerable areas using both sturdy parts of the body and a variety of standard and impromptu weapons.

Krav Maga emphasizes training under stressful conditions to prepare students for crisis conditions. There is an emphasis on aggression and survival as primary values of the art.

Beyond simple assault situations, Krav Maga includes a

Gross Motor Skills

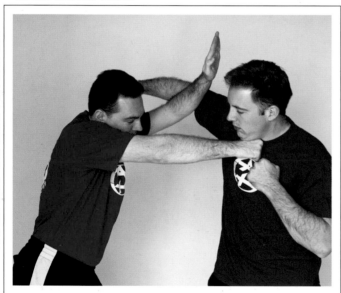

- Krav Maga is trained with an emphasis on gross motor skills rather than small, fine movements.

- In stressful situations you become adrenalized and cannot rely on fine movements. Krav Maga instead bases its approach on the skills we can use even under the most grueling conditions.

- Krav Maga training also includes methods that place you in an adrenalized state, so that you have experience performing under pressure.

Natural Human Reflexes

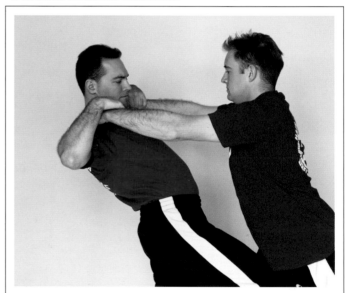

- Krav Maga techniques take advantage of existing reflexes that we all share.

- When we are choked, for example, the instinctive response is to bring our hands to our neck.

- By practicing a defense that begins with the reflexive movement, Krav Maga teaches skill that can be learned quickly and retained with a minimum of practice.

- The efficiency in Krav Maga's techniques is also highly visible in its training methods and conceptual approach.

significant portion of training for dealing with armed attackers. Students undergo extensive training in defending and disarming sticks, knives, handguns, long guns, and even grenades. Because of Krav Maga's military origin, it is a popular choice for military, LEO, and antiterrorism training.

Aggressive Defenses

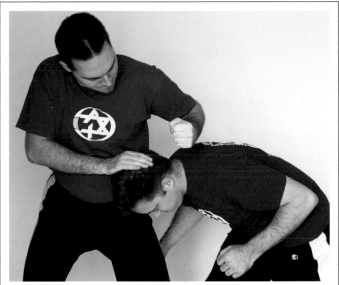

- Krav Maga emphasizes attacking the most vulnerable areas and in rapid succession. Strikes are thrown in heavy bunches, often targeting the groin, eye, and throat.

- Practitioners are trained to attack and defend in the shortest time possible, often beginning their counterattack while simultaneously defending the threat.

- Drills are done under stressful conditions to improve your ability to defend appropriately when agitated.

Emphasis on Practicality

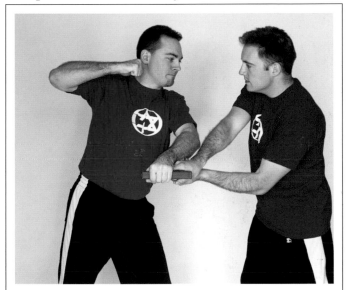

- Its techniques are quick and vicious. Krav Maga teaches you to respond immediately and aggressively.

- Krav Maga's techniques were put through extreme testing and real-world analysis as it was developed. It still undergoes evolution and revision.

- Owing to Krav Maga's training methods and use of natural reflexes, its skills can be built quickly. It's a great art for developing usable skills in a short period of time.

JEET KUNE DO
Bruce Lee's method of training adapts to any kind of fight or fighter

Jeet Kune Do (JKD), or "the way of the intercepting fist," is not a martial art but rather a training method designed to teach each individual student to adapt.

JKD training focuses first on self-preservation skills or the ability to survive assault in any of the ranges or phases where an individual may be forced to fight. After skill sets have been established in each of the major areas, students pursue their own unique path by studying their experiences using the tools they have learned and finding a unique combination that is most effective for them as individuals.

JKD does not have its own curriculum but instead offers training methods that allow students to learn skills from many styles. They might learn Thai, French, Chinese, Japanese, and American styles of kickboxing and then experiment with using these skills against each other until each student has a working knowledge of how he or she

Empty Hand Fighting

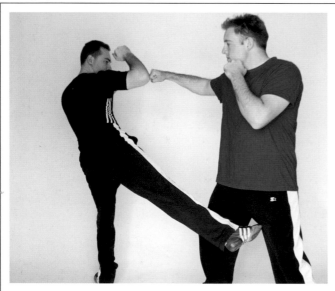

- Jeet Kune Do is a system of training methods that teaches the individual to adapt to any situation.

- Drawing its techniques from all sources, it emphasizes using the most efficient and effective tools for each range or phase of combat.

- Each JKD practitioner develops his own method, unique to his personality, body type, and experiences. JKD training provides the laboratory environment where each student can experiment and discover, through experience, what works for him.

Weapons Training

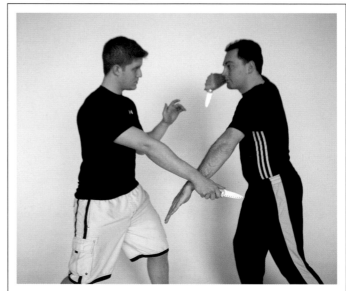

- Jeet Kune Do training involves the integration of weapons into all other areas, from kickboxing to ground fighting.

- Training includes weapon-versus-weapon and empty hand-versus-weapon situations. Each individual must have experience adapting to any situation.

- JKD training is often tied with the Filipino martial arts, which carry a long tradition of fighting using blades of all sizes.

personally can best use the various techniques and tools.

JKD training involves a process like this for all of the major areas of fighting, including striking, grappling, and weapons. Environmental concerns, complex situations, and much more are studied, experienced, and evaluated.

JKD was designed to coach the student through hundreds of hours of experience fighting against every kind of fighter in any imaginable situation so that the student will know with confidence how he or she can best approach that situation in a real fight. The result will be different for every individual because each person comes to the training with a different personality, body type, set of experiences, and life situation. Because of this fact, no two JKD practitioners will do things exactly alike because they themselves are not exactly alike.

Adapting to Any Situation

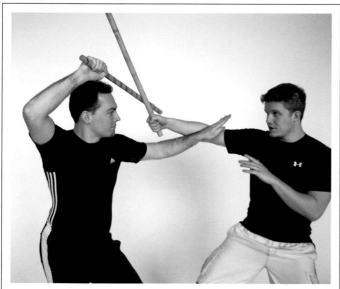

- Training in Jeet Kune Do involves boxing, kickboxing, trapping, clinching, and ground fighting. It investigates a variety of approaches from around the globe for each of these areas.

- Additionally it includes the study of blunt, flexible, edged, and projectile weapons in each of those areas.

- Training is also done in a variety of environments and in tough situations such as two-on-one and three-on-one fights against multiple attackers.

Finding a Unique Way

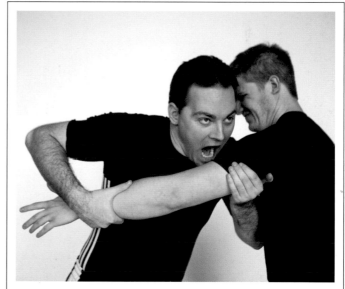

- After students are proficient in the various ranges and methods of fighting, they combine the techniques and tactics into a unique, personal synthesis that suits them individually.

- No area of training is left unobserved by JKD training. It is a long study, but it offers the most thorough experience possible.

- It takes many years of training for an individual to reach a high level of proficiency in all of JKD's areas of study.

BRAZILIAN JIU-JITSU

Control bigger and stronger attackers on the ground using a reinvention of Japanese Jiu-Jitsu

Popularized by its role in the growing sport of mixed martial arts, Brazilian Jiu-Jitsu (BJJ) has become the world's premier art for grappling and ground fighting.

Brought to South America in the early 1900s by a Japanese immigrant, Jiu-Jitsu went through decades of revision, testing, and evolution in Brazil to become its own unique

approach to the art and to fighting. Focused almost exclusively on ground fighting, BJJ offers a means of controlling a bigger, heavier, and stronger attacker by precise body positioning and the proper use of space and weight. Although it appears similar to wrestling, BJJ does not focus on the ability to pin the opponent but rather to catch him in a technique

Learning to Control

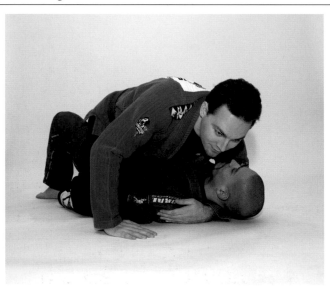

- Brazilian Jiu-Jitsu training focuses on the ground-fighting aspect of self-defense.

- Students learn to control an opponent who is bigger, heavier, and stronger by employing the most efficient use of their weight and strength.

- BJJ training also has a heavy focus on escaping someone's control, so they can hold you pinned on the ground only with difficulty.

- Because of its emphasis on technique over strength, BJJ is popular with men and women of all sizes.

Finishing a Fight

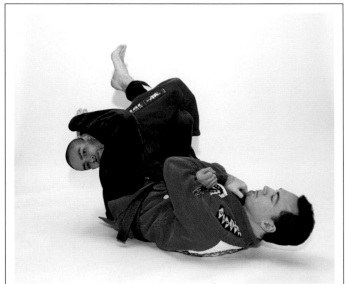

- The primary strategy of Brazilian Jiu-Jitsu is to take control of the opponent by establishing a superior position. The positions of BJJ typically involve taking control of the hips so that the center of gravity is dominated.

- From there the BJJ practi-

tioner seeks to end the fight by applying a technique that will break his opponent's arm or leg or choke him unconscious.

- These techniques, known as "submissions" in training, are the type that could incapacitate an attacker and end an assault.

that would cause grave injury, such as a broken arm or leg, in a real situation. These techniques are taught so that even a smaller, weaker practitioner could employ them successfully on an uncooperative aggressor.

One of the key elements of Brazilian Jiu-Jitsu's success is the emphasis on sparring against a resistant partner, which is called "rolling." In BJJ training rolling is a daily training method that allows students to determine their relative effectiveness against someone who tries to beat them. In some environments the partner may be allowed to strike at them or use other tactics that might be used in a real fight.

Equally important as its ability to teach control, Brazilian Jiu-Jitsu teaches students to escape pins, locks, chokes, and throws from their partners. Practitioners are expected to develop the ability to escape, even when pinned under a much bigger, stronger opponent who is not allowing them to move. Because of the enormous emphasis on applied skill against resistance, BJJ practitioners have a reputation for reaching exceptional skill levels within their art.

Using Leverage

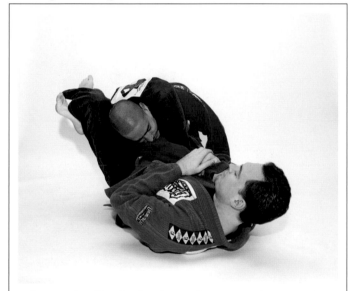

- Because Brazilian Jiu-Jitsu is intended to use a person's strength maximally, it features an emphasis on using the hips to move.

- The hips are surrounded by some of the largest, strongest muscles of the body, especially in women. BJJ teaches the student how to use that strength to overcome size or weight disparity or tremendous upper-body strength.

- BJJ develops dexterity and agility in the legs, so that they can be used to control an attacker or even choke him unconscious.

Safe and Humane

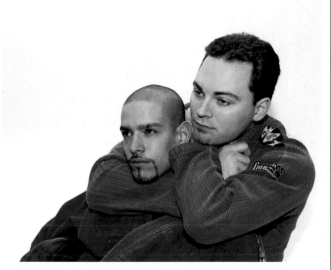

- Brazilian Jiu-Jitsu is popular for its emphasis on training methods that constantly test the student's ability to perform in realistic conditions.

- It is also hailed as a humane approach to fighting because it presents options for ending a conflict by putting your opponent to sleep or by using the threat of injury.

- In more dire situations, the techniques are effective at causing major injury to the joints, which can make it difficult for your attacker to continue the assault.

223

JUDO

Toss people around with Japan's gentle art for mutual welfare and benefit

Japan's art of judo is another modern martial art that offers particularly useful training for those interested in self-defense. By learning to wrestle with opponents, students develop strong balance and the ability to withstand and defeat attempts to take them to the ground and control them.

Developed around the turn of the twentieth century, judo is a modern combination of several older styles of Japanese jujitsu. As a result of strong and thoughtful organization, judo is taught with a universal curriculum, so students around the world learn the same skills in the same sequence.

Judo focuses primarily on the ability to throw one's opponent to the ground. The trips, takedowns, and throws of judo

Using the Hips

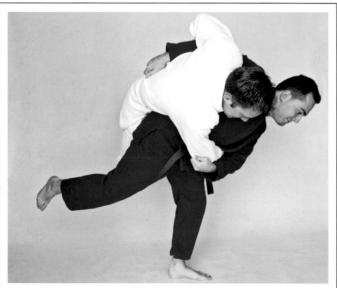

- Judo centers its action on the power of the hips for lifting and throwing.

- Modern judo is most commonly known for being an Olympic sport and for its visually stunning throws.

- Judo is a grappling art that does not typically train strikes. Judo schools teach a combination of throwing and takedown skills from the clinch as well as pinning skills on the ground.

- Judo also features some submission techniques in its adult classes.

Grappling and Throwing

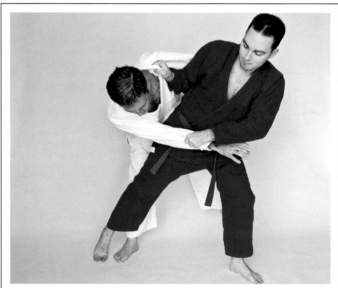

- Because judo technique is primarily focused on the use of the hips, it is a popular art for women.

- It also focuses on the principle of using the opponent's energies against him, which works well when fighting someone physically bigger or stronger.

- Training in judo provides you with hours of hands-on experience learning to keep your balance—and throw your attacker off balance.

- Much of judo is tested in competition-style training to ensure that the student can perform the skills on a noncompliant opponent.

are powerful techniques, reliant upon the use of the strong muscles of the hips rather than those of the upper body.

Similar to Brazilian Jiu-Jitsu, judo also has a ground-fighting component to its grappling. Although it is more restrictive than BJJ, their shared history makes the two arts similar in their techniques and principles.

Known today primarily as an Olympic sport, judo balances the traditional training methods, sport preparation, and character development elements that intertwine to make judo the unique art it is.

Maximum Efficiency

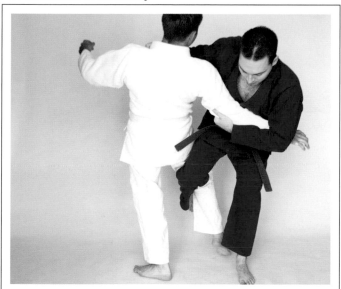

- One of the two most popular maxims at the heart of judo is maximum efficiency and minimum effort.

- Students are taught to make the most of their strength by developing precise technique to launch their opponents to the ground.

- Competitive training allows students to hone their technique and to develop the precise timing that will allow them to control their opponent effectively.

Mutual Welfare and Benefit

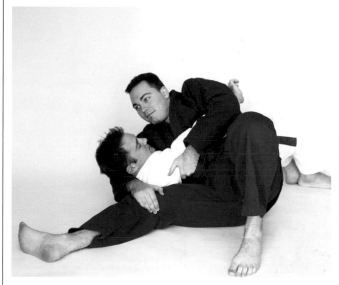

- Judo is one of the most popular martial arts in the country. Because judo was one of the first martial arts to land in the United States, it has had considerable time to establish deep roots and far-reaching branches across the country.

- Because of its broad reach and emphasis on community, judo is also often fairly inexpensive. This makes it accessible to many folks who might not be able to study martial arts otherwise.

BOXING

The sweet science stresses effective movement, footwork, and hands of steel

Boxing has been a part of the Western sport tradition for hundreds of years in various manifestations. Boxing's connection to the realm of fighting has never been questioned because of its obvious carryover in skills and technique.

Perhaps the most critical skills learned by boxers are those of movement and of defense. The ability to avoid, to evade, and to outflank an opponent who is trying to hit you is of immense value for self-defense. Whether the goal is to escape one opponent or many, there is no skill more coveted than that of good footwork and the ability to move quickly and easily to a safe distance and location.

Boxers develop the ability to see and defend punches as

Striking Power

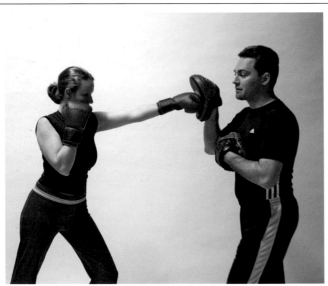

- Boxers develop the ability to throw lightning-fast, powerful punches with laser accuracy.

- For self-defense purposes, learning to hit well is essential. Boxing provides a fantastic structure and base for outstanding fighting abilities.

- The basic punches of boxing—the jab, cross, hook, and uppercut—form the foundation of solid striking with the hands.

- Boxers learn to use their body to generate massive amounts of power, so that they can strike with every ounce of muscle.

Movement and Defense

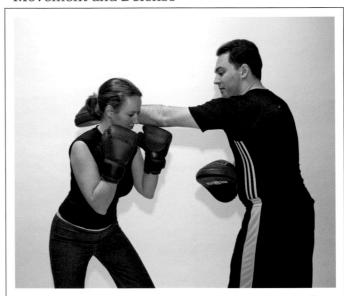

- Boxers train in the essential skills of moving and defending. Footwork is a major emphasis because it helps place you exactly where you need to be so you can hit without being hit.

- When it comes to defense, boxers learn to stop a punch—and also how to take one and keep fighting.

- Conditioning plays a major role, and the ability to weather punches is a critical asset.

well as the toughness and courage to continue if they are struck. Boxers develop a will to survive in the ring that translates appropriately to the realm of self-defense.

In the offensive realm, boxers develop a core set of punching tools that are fast, strong, and accurate. They devote endless hours to the perfection of these few techniques to master every subtlety of their application and timing in order to score dominating punches again and again even on skilled opponents.

Stick and Move

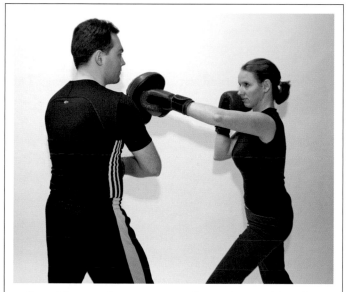

- One of the most important abilities that boxers develop is the ability to see punches coming, even in a fraction of a second.

- They train their awareness so that they can react in a split second to a strike headed their way.

- Boxers learn to hit and to move so that they are not hit in return. They perfect their timing and awareness to minimize risk to themselves while outstriking their opponents.

Fighting Fitness

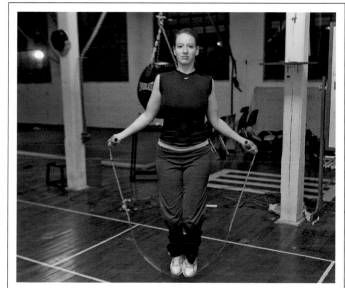

- Fitness is a major focus in boxing. Stamina and endurance play major roles in the training.

- It is not uncommon for boxers to run several miles a day in order to help develop cardiovascular endurance—as well as the muscular endurance of their legs for countless rounds of footwork and punching power.

- Many boxers run before starting their daily training. Boxers put themselves into top shape for their sport.

RECOMMENDED SCHOOLS

My School

Modern Self-defense Center, Middletown, CT

www.modernselfdefense.com

Since 2002 Modern Self-defense Center (MSDC) has been central Connecticut's hub for martial arts and self-defense training. MSDC offers Brazilian Jiu-Jitsu, Jeet Kune Do, boxe Francaise savate (French kickboxing), mixed martial arts, and a weekly free self-defense class.

Some of My Instructors

I welcome you to contact these excellent schools in order to train with them. I have nothing but the finest things to say about the training I have received from each of these institutions.

Harris Academy, San Diego, CA

www.royharris.com

Led by self-defense expert Roy Harris, the Harris Academy offers training in Bruce Lee's Jeet Kune Do, Filipino martial arts, Brazilian Jiu-Jitsu, Kalis Ilustrisimo, self-defense, Mixed Martial Arts, law enforcement defensive tactics, and kettlebells.

Krav Maga NYC, New York

www.kravmagainc.com

The Krav Maga Federation headquarters is led by master instructor Rhon Mizrachi. He and his staff teach and preserve authentic Krav Maga of the highest caliber.

Middletown Kenpo Karate Studio, Middletown, CT

www.mkks.com

Founded by Professor Lee Lowery, Middletown Kenpo Karate Studio (MKKS) offers training in Kenpo Karate and Modern Arnis. Instructors have taught programs to students of all ages since the 1970s.

Friends and Associates

These are schools that I personally recommend. I have trained with each of these instructors and encourage you to train with them if they are in your area.

BDB Martial Arts, Calgary, Alberta, Canada

www.bdbma.com

Head instructor Brian Bird has coached world champions, including his wife, Sheila Bird, in grappling and Brazilian Jiu-Jitsu. BDB Martial Arts is the home of many high-level competitors in grappling, Muay Thai kickboxing, and Mixed Martial Arts.

Nomad Brazilian Jiu-Jitsu, Sherbrooke, Quebec, Canada

www.nomadbjj.com

Nomad Brazilian Jiu-Jitsu is led by innovative head instructor Rich Martens. Rich has been training in martial arts since a young age and is a frequent guest at my school.

Roy Dean Academy, Bend, OR

www.roydeanacademy.com

Roy Dean leads a Brazilian Jiu-Jitsu academy with a rare flavor of traditional Japanese training.

Saunders Brazilian Jiu-Jitsu, Rochester, NY

www.saundersbjj.com

Saunders Brazilian Jiu-Jitsu is an excellent club led by head instructor Kyle Saunders. Kyle has been involved in BJJ for over fifteen years and is a skilled practitioner and instructor.

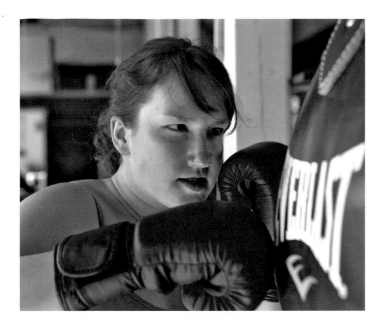
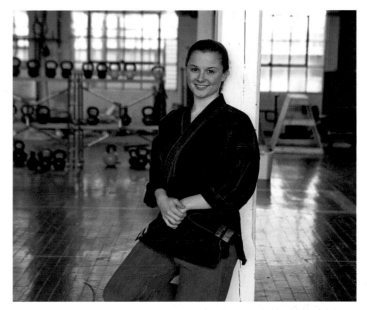
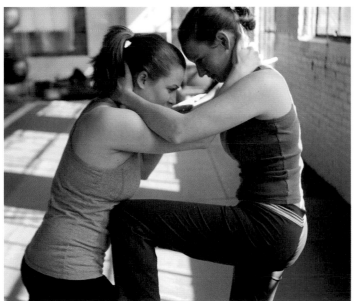
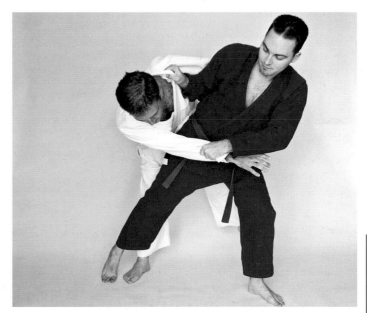

229

ORGANIZATIONS

Countless martial arts organizations are out there; these are some of the ones with which I have personal experience and gladly endorse.

Nontraditional Arts

Harris International Grappling Association
www.royharris.com

Harris International Jeet Kune Do/French, Filipino, and Indonesian Martial Arts Association
www.royharris.com

Krav Maga Federation
www.kravmagafederation.com

Traditional Arts

Budoshin Ju-Jitsu Yudanshakai
www.budoshin.com

International Modern Arnis Federation
www.modernarnis.net

New England Martial Arts Teachers Association

Judo has three major organizations in the United States:

United States Judo Association
www.usja-judo.org

United States Judo Federation
www.usjf.com

USA Judo
www.usjudo.org

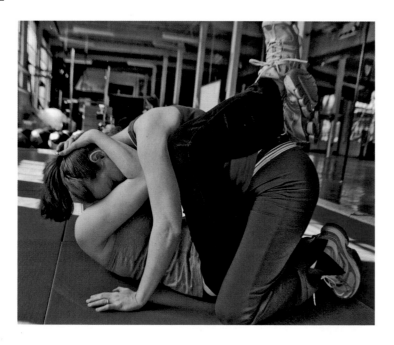

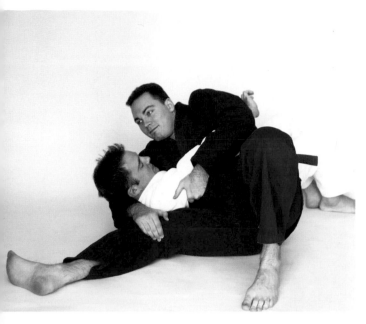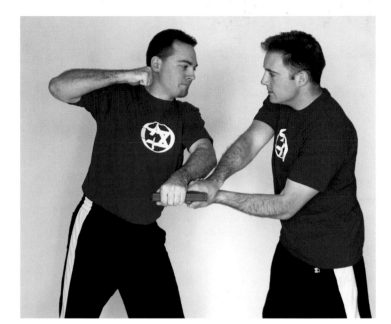

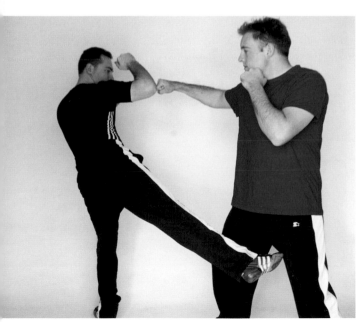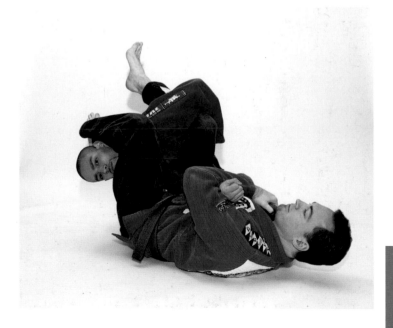

231

EQUIPMENT & TRAINING GEAR

Here are some established equipment providers for martial arts and self-defense equipment. I recommend the products made by these companies for your protection or training use.

Weapons and Self-defense Equipment

ASP
www.asp-net.com

Bud K
www.budk.com

Cold Steel
www.coldsteel.com

Training Equipment

Budovideos
www.budovideos.com

Century
www.centurymartialarts.com

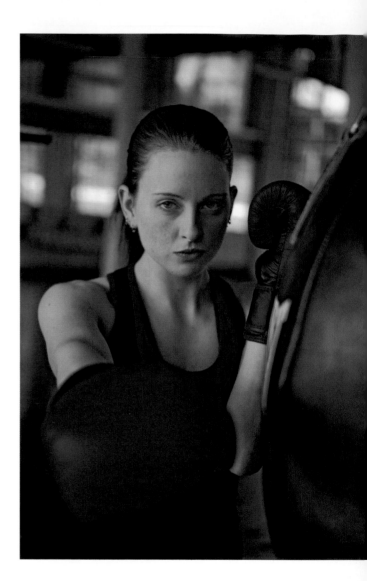

RESOURCES

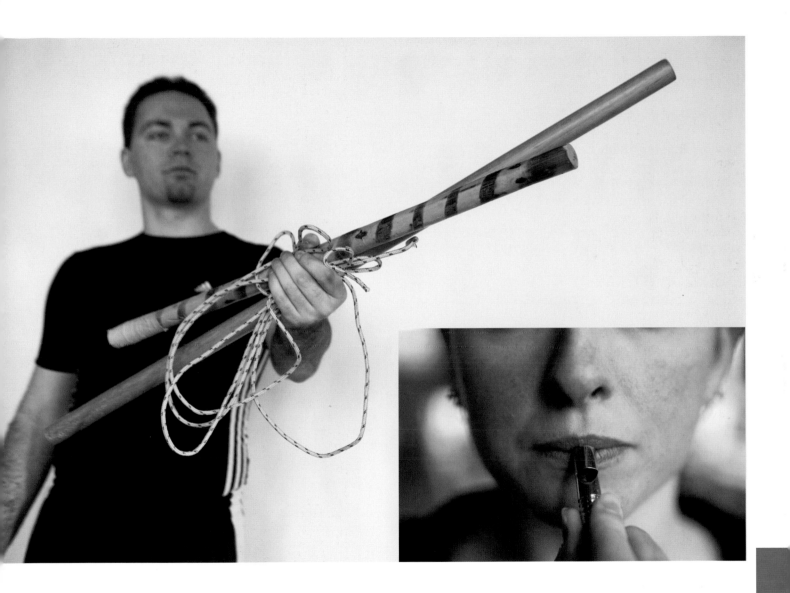

FOR FURTHER READING

Books

Disaster Planning

Emergency: This Book Will Save Your Life by Neil Strauss. It Books, 2009

Reading Faces and Body Language

Knack Body Language: Techniques on Interpreting Nonverbal Cues in the World and Workplace by Aaron Brehove. Knack, 2010

Telling Lies: Clues to Deceit in the Marketplace, Politics, and Marriage by Paul Ekman. W. W. Norton & Company, 2009

Unmasking the Face: A Guide to Recognizing Emotions from Facial Expressions by Paul Ekman and Wallace V. Friesen. Malor Books, 2003

Self-defense versus Weapons

Krav Maga: How to Defend Yourself Against Armed Assault by Imi Sde Or and Eyal Yanilov. Frog Books, 2001

Magazines

Black Belt Magazine
www.blackbeltmagazine.com

Ultimate MMA
www.ultimategrapplingmag.com

E-Journal of Jujutsu
www.jujutsujournal.com

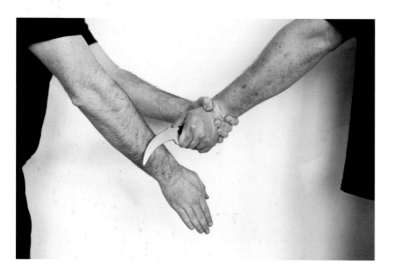

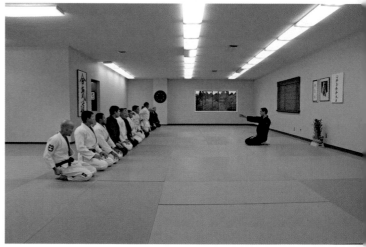

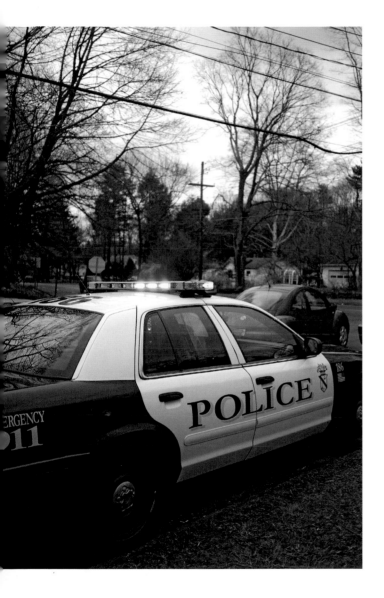

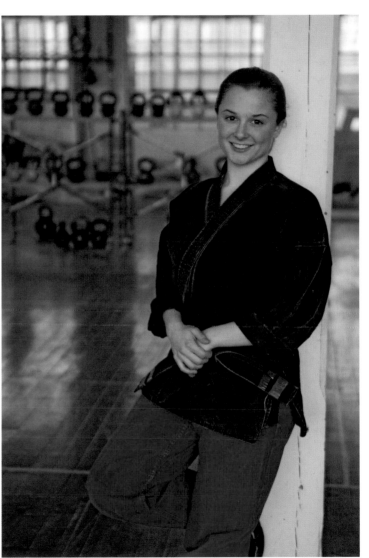

WEB SITES

Training Martial Arts

Mixed Martial Arts.com Forums

www.mixedmartialarts.com

Discussion forums sorted by martial art and geographical region and many Q&A forums led by experts.

Health and Fitness

Dragondoor—Hard Style Kettlebell Training

www.dragondoor.com

Pavel Tsatsouline's organization leads the field in hard-style kettlebell training, as well as strength and flexibility development.

Functional Movement Systems

www.functionalmovement.com

Gray Cook and Lee Burton have developed tools for evaluating and assessing an individual's movement patterns in order to prevent injury and improve athletic performance.

Dr. Mark Cheng—Kettlebells Los Angeles

www.kettlebellslosangeles.com
www.kettlebellslosangeles.blogspot.com

Dr. Mark Cheng, head of Kettlebells Los Angeles, is a highly sought expert in movement and joint health, especially as it applies to martial arts and self-defense training. He carries my highest personal recommendation.

Postassault Management

National Domestic Violence Hotline

www.ndvh.org
(800) 799-SAFE

National Hopeline Network—24-Hour Hotline

www.hopeline.com
(800) SUICIDE

Rape, Abuse, and Incest National Network

www.rainn.org
(800) 656-HOPE

Sexual Assault Support Services—24-Hour Crisis and Support Hotline

www.sass-lane.org
(800) 788-4727

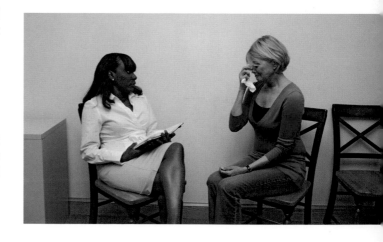

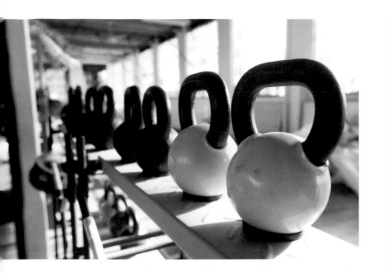

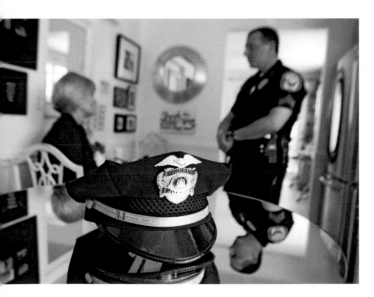

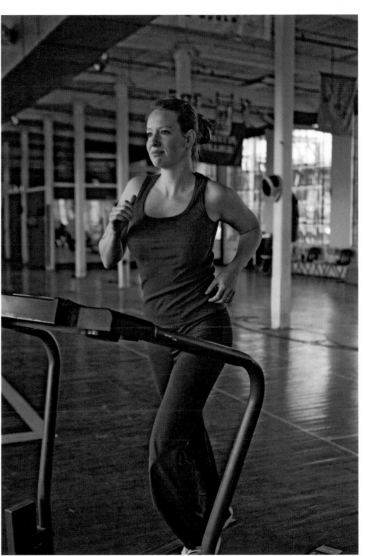

GLOSSARY

Armlock: A technique that pits the leverage of the trunk of the body against the wrist, elbow, or shoulder joints, breaking or dislocating the joint.

Blunt weapons: *See* **Impact weapons.**

Boxing: Centuries-old sport and martial art that focuses on the use of punches and their defenses in order to defeat an opponent.

Boxing range: A distance of one arm's length away, where punches can be throw to full extension and will reach their target.

Brazilian Jiu-Jitsu: Martial art and sport that focuses on ground fighting. Emphasizes the use of leverage and positioning to control bigger, stronger attackers using minimal strength. Does not include striking, instead favoring submission techniques including chokes, armlocks, and leglocks.

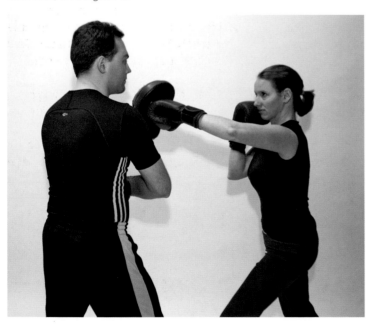

Centerline: The primary axis of the body, from the top of the head down through the center of the torso.

Choke: A technique that applies pressure to the neck, diminishing either the passage of air to the lungs or blood to the brain. Sometimes subdivided into chokes versus strangulations.

Clinch: A phase of fighting in which one or both participants attempt to wrestle for control of the other while standing.

Clinch range: The closest distance for fighting while on the feet—both parties are almost or completely body to body and are using or attempting some form of control.

Closed guard: A position used in Brazilian Jiu-Jitsu in which the defender lies on her back and wraps her legs around her kneeling aggressor's midsection. The ankles are crossed, thus "closing" the guard.

Edged weapon: Any sharp implement used as a weapon. Commonly refers to knives, swords, or other blades.

Flexible weapon: A weapon, including rope, chain, fishing line, or whips, that can bend, often used either for impact or entanglement.

Grappling: Wrestling for control through pulling and pushing or the body.

Ground fighting, ground range: A phase of fighting in which one or both parties are seated or lying on the ground. Most commonly one party is applying his weight to the other in an attempt to control him.

Guard: A position popularized by Brazilian Jiu-Jitsu in which one party, lying on his back or seated, controls the other person (on top of him) using a combination of his arms and legs.

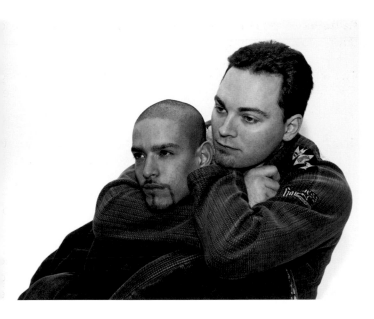

Hammer strike: A blow using the underside of the fist, along the pinky side of the hand.

Impact weapons: Weapons or other implements used for striking that are used for blunt trauma. Impact weapons often create advantages in distance or strength of the material: sticks, bats, brass knuckles, and so forth.

Jeet Kune Do: Created by Bruce Lee, a system of training methods that trains individuals to pursue experiences that will help them adapt to any combative situation.

Judo: A Japanese martial art and Olympic sport that focuses on throwing the opponent to the ground and applying a pin or submission.

Kickboxing range: The distance from which punches and kicks can be thrown to full extension but will still reach their target.

Krav Maga: An Israeli martial art of military origins that focuses on aggressive, easily learned skills for common threats.

Mount: A position in ground fighting popularized by Brazilian Jiu-Jitsu in which one party controls the other by kneeling over his partner's midsection.

Open guard: A ground-fighting position in which one party, seated or lying down, controls the other by pushing on the front of his body with his hands, elbows, feet, and knees. Compare with the **closed guard.**

Projectile weapons: Weapons that fire their ammunition at someone. They include firearms, bow and arrows, crossbows, and aerosolized weapons such as pepper spray and Mace.

Side: A pinning position popular in Judo and Brazilian Jiu-Jitsu in which one party holds the other to the ground, chest to chest, with both legs on the same side of the pinned partner's body. Sometimes called "side mount," "side control," "100 kilos," "Yoko Shiho Gatame," and so forth. (I have called it "the side" in this book to avoid confusion.)

Sportive martial art: Martial art in which the primary training methods revolve around sport practices of sparring and competition.

Traditional martial art: Martial art in which sporting practices are secondary (or unused) and emphasis is instead on character development and form for the sake of artistic development.

Trapping: Techniques in which a hand or leg is temporarily pinned in place in order to create a clear path to hit or grab, typically on the body's centerline.

Trapping range: The distance at which trapping techniques can be employed.

INDEX

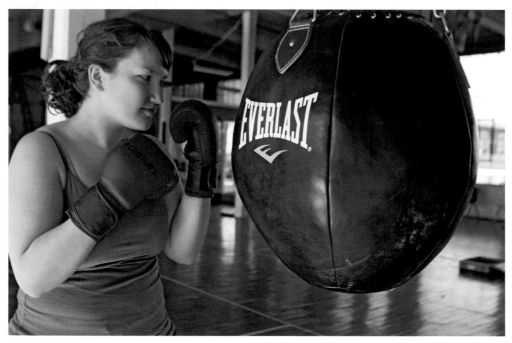

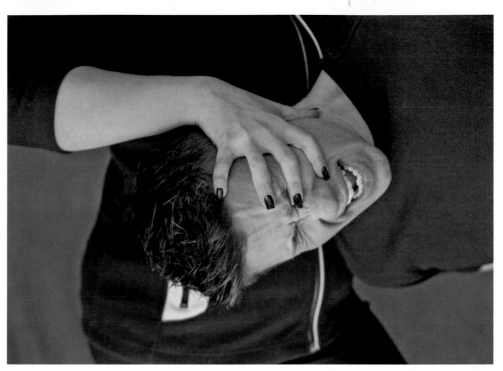

241

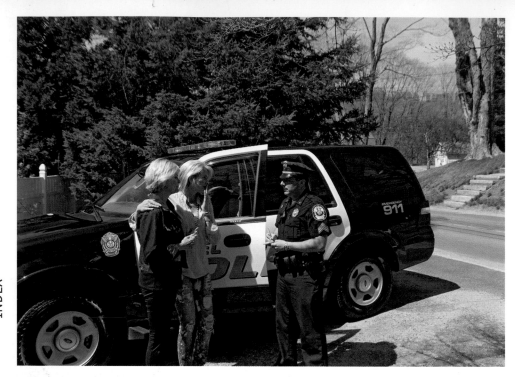

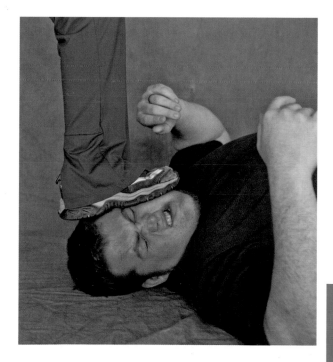

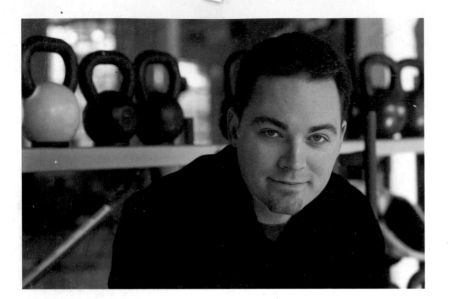

About the Author

Chris Wright-Martell, who has been practicing and teaching Brazilian Jiu-Jitsu and Jeet Kune Do for many years, heads the Modern Self-Defense Center in Middletown, Connecticut, which specializes in contemporary self-defense training. Chris and his self-defense techniques have been featured on major media outlets including ABC news. Visit him at modernselfdefense.com.

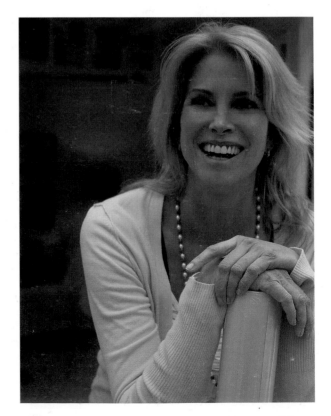

About the Photographer

Kristen Jensen became a photo journalist after twenty-five years of modeling for the Willamena and Ford agencies, and is today a leading lifestyle and portrait photographer, distinguished for the modern, candid style she has brought to capturing the elusive beauty of everything from weddings to the latest trends in the fashion modeling industry. She lives in Bethel, Connecticut. Visit her at kristenjensen.com.